SCARS TO PEARLS

SCARS TO PEARLS

A Medical Healing and Spiritual Journey Through
the Phases of Malignant Melanoma Stage IIIA
Skin Cancer with Micro-Metastasis.

LITA M. WORTHINGTON RNC, RNP
OB-GYN, REINFERTILITY NURSE PRACTITIONER

ELM HILL

A Division of
HarperCollins Christian Publishing

www.elmhillbooks.com

SCARS TO PEARLS

Published in Nashville, Tennessee, by Elm Hill, an imprint of Thomas Nelson. Elm Hill and Thomas Nelson are registered trademarks of HarperCollins Christian Publishing, Inc.

Elm Hill titles may be purchased in bulk for educational, business, fund-raising, or sales promotional use. For information, please e-mail SpecialMarkets@ThomasNelson.com.

All Scripture quotations, unless otherwise indicated, are taken from the Holy Bible, New International Version', NIV'. Copyright © 1973, 1978, 1984, 2011 by Biblica, Inc.' Used by permission of Zondervan. All rights reserved worldwide. www.Zondervan.com. The "NIV" and "New International Version" are trademarks registered in the United States Patent and Trademark Office by Biblica, Inc.'

Scripture Notations are from the following sources

Thin Line Bible, NIV (1996). Zondervan Publishing

Referenced Authors within this Book include:

Stanley, Charles F. (2017). The Charles F. Stanley Life Principles Bible, C. F. Stanley (Ed). Thomas Nelson

Young, Sarah (2004). Jesus Calling, Enjoying Peace in His Presence, S. Young (Ed). Nashville, TN by Thomas Nelson

Morgan, Robert J. (2016). The Strength You Need, R. J. Morgan (Ed). Nashville, TN by W Publishing Group, Imprint of Thomas Nelson

Collins, Francis S. (2006). The Language of God, F. S. Collins (Ed). New York, NY, Free Press a Division of Simon & Schuster, Inc.

NIV Women's Devotional New Testament with Psalms & Proverbs (1993). Zondervan Publishing

Referenced Institution Mentioned in this Book

Stanford Health Care, Stanford Cancer Center

Library of Congress Cataloging-in-Publication Data

Library of Congress Control Number: 2018948245

ISBN 978-1-595558237 (Paperback)
ISBN 978-1-595558282 (Hardbound)
ISBN 978-1-595558497 (eBook)

I Dedicate this Book to;

My husband Scott ~
God brought us together
Without your love and unfailing support
My life would be empty
You are my life
Thank you for loving me

To Lindsay, Matthew, Hawkeye, Easton, Kendyl, Daniel,
Karrington, and Reagan
How blessed am I
To have you all be my rock ~ when I needed you most
I cherished all my boo-boo kisses and squishes
Thank you for loving me

To my entire family, Pastor and friends
How I have appreciated all the love
Thoughts and prayers this past year
You have meant so much to me and I am humbled
Thank you for loving me

To my entire team of physicians and staff
Your knowledge and confidence
Allowed me to trust you with my care

Please know I'm grateful and love you all

INTRODUCTION

Walk with me on a journey toward Heaven

"Our journey toward Heaven begins with each step we take here on this earth. At times we chose a path that seems lost or off track. We are constantly redirecting or not. Our life's journey does not mean we will never experience sin, failure, frustration, hardships or trials. A life without pain, sin, trials or failure is simply not a guarantee. Our trek can be on rugged terrain with steep climbs and unsteady footing. But our time spent in His Word, with His Gift, His Riches to us will strengthen and mature our trust in Him. It is with trust in Christ Jesus that sheds light unto our path, eases our trek, and stabilizes our footing. Then our journey toward Heaven will be filled with Peace to guard our hearts and minds, always. It will always be through Him who gives us strength to continue the climb. Even with a mature faith and love for our Lord, our challenges on this earth continue. But it is the hope of salvation and life eternal with Him that help during these trials. I'm counting on it. We cannot know the strength of our faith until it has been tested. Even during our trials, He is watching and waiting for us to seek Him out. It is with prayer and a thankful heart which will grab His attention. For He is always watching and waiting for us to invite Him in. He will hold us by our right hand and He will meet us in the quietness of our soul."

I wrote the opening notation when I found out I had malignant melanoma skin cancer, Stage I, for the second time. This was late January of 2017 and I had just made it past my third year of being clear, without reoccurrence from my first diagnosis back in November 2013. *No big deal*, many of those who have had melanoma skin cancer stage I before would think. *Get it excised and move on with life*. This is what I also thought at first. But it was the news of cancer having made its ghostly way into my lymph nodes that redirected my plans for the year. Suddenly I was Stage III A, and the unexpected had occurred. How did this happen?

One of the major contributors to skin cancer is sun exposure. I have lived a very sun-exposed life, having participated in competitive outdoor athletic activities of tennis and swimming at a very young age, and still do. I also experienced life on a tropical island for about six years and, for the past fifty, sunny California has been my home. This coupled with a significant family history of skin cancer, my personal history with ALL three of the various skin cancers, and the medical provider in me (OB-GYN nurse practitioner) motivated me in part to bring additional awareness to skin cancer and all that surrounds it. The good news is I do not have to reinvent the wheel here.

There are many experts already leading the charge on skin cancer research. We have excellent cancer research institutions in the United States and I was fortunate to literally stumble into one of them. The health institution I crossed paths with has been recognized and earned top designation from the National Cancer Institute (NCI) for its broad scope of research, in which they are known to be a leader in breakthrough treatments. They were one of only forty-nine top cancer centers to receive such recognition. A prestigious and well deserved acknowledgement. The multidisciplinary care within the entire department was executed seamlessly. I did not know any of this with my first appointment. It was by chance that Stanford Medicine, Dermatology Clinic and Cutaneous Oncology, is where my story begins. I have been appreciative of all the medical expertise within this department and the attention I have received during my recent diagnosis. Which is why they deserve recognition in this book. However, I will not be mentioning any of my team of physicians by name.

I have learned so much about skin cancer and felt provoked to share the most accurate facts from current information available regarding the risks associated with it. To receive care from well-respected and world-renowned leaders in the area of dermatology was my good fortune. I will be sharing a broad overview of current information on skin cancer and all that goes with it, in respect to my journey.

With my recurrent diagnosis, I have had excellent resources made available to me as I wandered again into the skin cancer arena. But a person usually doesn't just go research skin cancer, unless they have been diagnosed with it. So in trying to cope or deal with this new health challenge, I preferred to reach for spiritual encouragement and, in doing so, I experienced a spiritual revival. I thought perhaps in sharing my personal experience with this dual awareness which would infuse my life this past year, in the form of a book, it would reach more people. People who may not have otherwise given **skin cancer** or Christianity a second thought.

I am writing as a patient now. An awkward position for a provider to experience, as I am the one who is used to examining, diagnosing, and formulating a treatment plan. Now, I feel vulnerable and exposed. I began journaling for spiritual therapy at first. But as I proceeded through one phase of treatment to the next, with such raw emotion I began including in my journaling the medical experience through the different diagnostic phases and surgeries I would eventually progress through. With the end goal of being cancer-free. I journaled almost the complete year in regards to malignant melanoma and all that went with that diagnosis for me. There came a moment, many months later, August in fact, in which I would feel compelled to write this book, share my experience, and bring a heightened awareness to the universally number one diagnosed, reported, and treated cancer—skin cancer.

I chose to keep a chronological order to the process of dealing with this diagnosis and all those that surrounded it as the year unfolded. I felt passionate to include more skin cancer awareness so you will find I address all skin cancers, the serious threat they can pose if ignored, as well as who is at risk. I review only my treatment options, as treatment plans need to be individualized from patient to patient, with so many factors to take into consideration that are between you and your physician. All my surgeries are detailed, including: shave biopsies, complete reexcision surgery, sentinel lymph node dissection biopsy (SLN), complete axillary lymph node dissection (ALND), and Mohs surgery (from the physician, Frederic E. Mohs; is a microscopically controlled surgery used to treat common types of skin carcinoma). Preventative measures with mole mapping and routine skin self-exam and, in my case, the additional potential complications in dealing with lymphedema are outlined. Helpful hints with a common-sense approach in regards to lymphedema, signs and symptoms, lymphatic massage exercises, importance of keeping up your immune system, when there has been an insult to it, are included. I will share which immunizations and vaccinations to consider if over the age of fifty, especially if immune-compromised, but at a minimum should warrant further discussion with your physician.

I do not include the staging for melanoma cancer in this book, as this is an area you as the patient must really understand. If the guidelines change, your physician will be able to better discuss with you what stage cancer you are in. Staging does require a collaborative effort of many different professionals besides your managing physician. The pathologist, radiologist and cancer registrar provide valuable staging information to your physician (s), who is the only one who has routine access to your personal history and all your pertinent information (biopsies, imaging studies, procedures, surgical findings) regarding your initial diagnosis. So with the entire picture in front of them, they take the lead in staging for a cancer in a patient.

The skin cancer topics or related facts will be set in **black bold print** and sprinkled throughout as my story unfolds. I will add a **Medical Pearl**, which could be a fact or medical suggestion to pay additional attention to, and this will be emphasized and set in **black bold print** as well.

I came to recognize that as I progressed from one area of specialty within the dermatology department to another, I was relying completely on their expertise and a flawless execution of it to promote an optimum outcome for me. Out of fear, my expectations were extremely high for my team of physicians and staff to provide care and execute the treatment plan—near perfectly. Isn't this what most patients expect from doctors—asking, do I really have the best? Then I realized while I am frightened going through this—whatever 'this' is and whatever outcome awaits me—it is an unfair expectation to have on them. But I had never met any of them before, nor did I know their skill level or reputation within their field. Of course they will try their best: they've taken an oath to do so, but they are not God. I needed to rely on my faith in Jesus above all else. He who is so much more qualified and will oversee my team of physicians for me. He is the Chief of Staff during all this, so to speak. So I would take the expectation off them and place it in the power of my prayer for them to execute their part to the best of their ability, as I transitioned through the phases of tackling this cancer. I can appreciate the fact we are all human, and I would soon recognize God has blessed some people with amazing, exceptional skills. I had just crossed paths with some of them and was extremely thankful I had.

In the months of pain and challenges, reaching for spiritual encouragement and journaling as the days, weeks, and months would pass, a spiritual awakening occurred, which was more powerful and unlike anything I have ever experienced. As the months unfolded, it began to stir a passion within me for writing this book. The Holy Spirit, definitely making His presence known to me throughout this journey, became my fuel and the driving force that would spark the idea. Could I merge these two topics—bring heightened awareness to skin cancer as I journey through its phases, *plus* incorporate how I came to be in a relationship with my Creator during this cancer challenge? I certainly could not write one topic without the other, because these two experiences were so tightly woven together within me as a whole. They were fused as my daily walk throughout the year. I will remember how and why my journey through malignant melanoma skin cancer, with all the scars serving as a constant reminder to me, would become a trek I will be forever thankful for.

I decided to write this semibiography in chronologic timeline as well while I progressed through the realm of my spiritual walk, appointments, surgeries, treatments, and recovery trying to become cancer-free. In trying to understand exactly what my faith means to me, I pulled from various sources and meditated on the truths of His promises in the quiet stillness of the mornings. I chose from a variety of resources, especially the NIV Bible, and when scripture is quoted, it will appear *italicized*. I have included very briefly a consolidated version of the history of the Bible, as I needed to try and understand where this all began. My thoughts on the definition of "faith," "trust," and The Holy Trinity as defined by me I reveal. I listened to online ministry, read daily devotionals, and a couple of well-written books. One book was written by a pastor, the other by a scientist/geneticist. I will share my spiritual thoughts, how I found myself in a relationship with God, and some past memories, which is why this reads like a biography, as it contributes to who I am. I find I must share my spiritual thoughts, visions/dreams, or **Spiritual Pearls** also, that occurred both past and present. How I deepened my faith, learned to pray, how you can pray, and several moments in which the Holy Spirit made His presence known to me during this cancer trial, which will have a title ***Holy Spirit Moment,*** both will be in ***italicized black bold print.***

Then there was an amazing experience my daughter and I shared the day of my 'big surgery,' which was life-altering for her, me, and many who pondered it long enough to see God had orchestrated the entire event. In one single moment, which took years in the making, He showed us the wonder of His Mercy. This experience surrounding my 'big surgery' day, slowly over time is what truly sparked the idea to write this and share it as written testimony. I believe it to be a testimony of His Word, being the Truth. We first sought Him out in prayer, we listened and because of His grace, He willingly answered us, as He often does, in visions or dreams. All of which will be mentioned in more detail as it would unfold before me. Each day I was discovering a spiritual yearning I never knew I had. As I spent time on the Bible getting to know Him over the months, He graced me with courage, strength, and hope to tackle all that awaited me. You will see how He allowed me to witness the Holy Spirit's presence off and on through phases in my recovery and provided strength in my setbacks. I would not be disappointed in my time spent with Him. You will not either. This was my chosen meditation or yoga for my mind, which gave me strength and hope throughout all my medical challenges and setbacks. But I am still only human.

I fueled my mind with scripture almost daily and over time in the maturing of my faith. I discovered what my new friend was all about. He unveiled something new to me daily. In time, I turned my faith into complete trust in Him. This complete trust in Him showered me with inner peace as my reward. His Perfect Peace. A peace that would calm my racing heart and mind. I found this inner peace provided me with the strength I needed to get through the challenge of the day, as some days were much more difficult than others. I will share scripture that helped restore my energy, nourish my soul, and provided the courage I would rely on in the midst of this trek. He would become my companion when I felt alone. I was merely a believer, and my life transformed as I welcomed being in a relationship with my God. His Truth provided all the hope I needed. But not 'hope' in the sense of 'I hope I get well soon,' or 'I hope it's true and there is a Heaven,' or even 'I hope I am right'; instead, it is with the 'Hope' of His Promise to all of us who love Him. A life everlasting with Him. My belief in my Maker is what sustains me and brings the greatest joy to my life. I recognize and accept this extraordinary gift that exists by faith alone. Something that our five senses cannot even confirm. It has been a choice for any of us to take advantage of, since His death on the cross was when *every single failure disappeared*. The same choice we ALL get to make now and in the future, until God calls us home.

I was also learning the meaning of patience as the hours, days, weeks, and months unfolded. I have a Type -A personality, so while recovering, sitting still all day long is difficult. However, as the days and weeks would pass, I began to get excited for what He was about to do. Day after day and week after week, as I would sit and read, and it took me several months before I realized I had discovered trusting Him completely meant 'without question' also. I began to trust in His plan for me no matter what. In case He doesn't move those mountains or chose to heal me, *His Promise is worth whatever challenge awaits me.* My desire was to stay in His Will. With His Grace and all my baby steps, I was experiencing growth and maturing of my faith, which brought me great joy during a significant trial in my life. I would gradually view all of my scars as my newfound pearls. At times I still cannot believe I have experienced this journey. I certainly did not welcome this trial, for my emotions would get the better of me at times as I share it all with you here. Until I saw how He equipped me to persevere through it, and He never left my side.

As you read on, I give a small Christian bio and share my first religious memory at the age of six or seven. It was extremely powerful and only as I wrote this book did I recall the details. The resources I gravitated towards and read on an almost daily basis were inspirational to me and led me to parts of scripture that would address my spectrum of emotions. I would recommend reading all of them. My emotional lability was very raw and the intensity at times was overwhelming and uncomfortable. It was a strong driving force, and I was committed to stay in His Word because I needed to. Even after months in prayer and journaling, I realized I never once prayed or bargained for a cure. It never even occurred to me. My only desire was to stay in His Will. After months meditating on His Word, my faith was gaining momentum. He continued to provide the strength along the way, and every single day for me.

Throughout my years as a Christian, I have experienced visions/dreams in the dark of the night. I do not include these to coerce you into believing for it is my walk, but they seem to have pertinence as I write this bio so I include some of them. I know this must occur to other people as well; I hear it often. Some of the visions/dreams have been uplifting and comforting, others dark and disturbing. I will share an extremely personal moment my daughter experienced while I was in surgery and the impact it had on my husband's family. I think it will prove emotional as we shared this moment with family and recognize the comfort that followed, convinced that our God is a merciful God and full of Grace.

This past year, which was filled with approximately fifty appointments both locally and at Stanford, two surgeries, hospitalization and therapies, life manages to continue. There will be the 'firsts' I discover that I cannot do as well, or partake of, as I try and adjust to a 'new normal' for my life. I will share family life and a family crisis with the sudden death of the matriarch of the family during my recovery. The stressors in life do not lie solely with our health challenges but also with work, family, and everything else on our plate. It can all seem overwhelming and cast doubts as to when any form of normalcy will return. Only when the 'new normal' is welcomed and feels natural again will our focus change for the better. You don't realize the months or even years this may take.

My journaling continues as I wait and ponder my options. But in considering my next steps with my diagnosis, I noticed *fear* beginning to loom within me. It seemed like it would take forever to make the final decision in my treatment plan. Where would this untraveled road I was about to embark on lead me? I needed to find courage, strength, and hope to move forward, as I knew I could not muster up the strength or courage on my own. No way. As a provider we need to exude confidence in our skills, diagnosis, and treatment plans for our patients. That is how I practiced anyway. Now as a patient, I will forever be aware of the ripple effect of worry, concern, and fear that my patients can have 'awaiting what is next' after a challenging diagnosis is delivered. I recall trying to reassure patients 'not to worry'; it seems almost insensitive now. Even when I am so confident in the potential outcome, it just seems insensitive. Some people will worry no matter what. The mind is the hardest thing to control and God knew this when He made us. I'm thinking so we would look to Him first with all our concerns.

I absolutely cannot imagine trying to tackle this on my own, especially when there is a way to find encouragement and hope that will provide the strength I now need. I know there are many people who have done so on their own. How? It must be so frightfully difficult. My faith was being tested, and I followed the pull of His power within my soul. I will share my own spiritual thoughts along the way through my various trials. This focus is what would shed the light on my path for what awaited me. God had a hand in this. I will witness the presence of the Holy Spirit on many occasions, and through almost each phase as I dealt with this challenge. I recognize all of this was a 'Gift' to me from God.

News of micrometastasis to my lymph nodes occurred in early March 2017, after I underwent a diagnostic procedure called lymphoscintigraphy or sentinel lymph node mapping. More options would need to be discussed following this new diagnosis. More surgery, diagnostic testing, blood work, and possibly a chemo-like infusion treatment called immunotherapy, partaking in a drug trial, and every-three-month skin checks could be my reality. The risk of melanoma spreading to other areas in the body can be a devastating and life-threatening cancer.

For those who are reading this book and have recently been diagnosed with cancer, I know you are scared; I certainly was. Because in the beginning when you first hear the news, you immediately wonder, 'How is this all going to end?' The journey has only just begun and we are already wondering how it's all going to play out. I know all the questions you are asking yourself, for I am the patient now and my perspective has changed. I can feel the uncertainty of your courage and strength to proceed through the demands of appointments, diagnostic testing, surgeries, pain, and treatments. I know the tears you will wipe quietly away from your cheek in the middle of the night when you can't sleep or when you are simply all alone, afraid, in pain, or discouraged. I can feel your heart pounding so loud that certainly anyone standing next to you must hear it also. Your mind is spinning with worry from all the 'what ifs.' Then there is the protective nature we have as a mother or father, to keep a brave appearance when we are around our loved ones, children (grown or not they are still our children), friends, but the fear of the unknown remains ever so real. I know your raw emotions, from concern, worry, discouragement, sadness, fear, pain, fatigue, loneliness, and exhaustion, just to name a few.

We often associate the word 'cancer' with end-of-life situations. It is a very hard word to hear for the first time. But even with all the uncertainty of the future, the hope for a positive outcome is always on the table. There can be 'hope' in every situation. Never lose hope. Positive thinking and hope should be in your treatment plan. Remember in the midst of all your fears there can be elation and thankfulness. Good news does happen. It can be felt deep in the soul, and it can be fueled by faith.

As I complete this introduction, I am nine months clear, with status posttreatment by choosing the surgical route of complete axillary lymph node dissection for malignant melanoma stage III, with micrometastasis to the lymph. I have had three brain MRIs and three PET scans that have all returned negative. This is all good news and puts me eleven months out from the original surgery, which took me from stage I to stage III overnight.

This was my second melanoma stage I diagnosis, but something was different. There would be options to discuss, as my overall family history and personal health history needed to be considered. I had a strong feeling that I couldn't ignore. After much dialogue with my team of physicians at Stanford, my family, but especially my dermatologist who suspected melanoma again to begin with, I chose to stay proactive. I have maintained an aggressive approach, which isn't for everyone, and diligently keep my follow-up appointments. I have had setbacks because of my proactive approach, but remain thankful I did, because the chance of malignant melanoma stage I cancer being in the lymph nodes at all was less than four to six percent. Nine months out and three scans later, I finally feel like I can breathe a little deeper, sleep a little sounder, and laugh a little louder.

Such great news came in the beginning of December, my absolute favorite month of the year. Just yesterday in fact, as I lunched with my mother and youngest sister, December 22, 2017, I said; "*I would go through this challenge all over again, because it was during THIS trial in my life that He grabbed my attention.*" This intimacy with my Maker I recognize as a Gift to me. A Gift of Grace and Hope that we unwrapped together. As I slowly and gently untied the ribbon and carefully opened this Gift, He would extend His hand and unveil inside a Promise. His Promise to be there for all who call Him by name. He walked with me. He talked with me. He sat with me. He had my right hand and provided the strength for my day, and it was always just enough. I was never alone. He carried my burdens, as I felt them lifted on occasion, and I will never let go of His hand.

In sharing my story, I must share a part of my life that includes where I came from and who I am spiritually, personally, and professionally. I had no idea my journey through this challenge would lead to this writing of my story. I certainly wasn't expecting the growth I would experience as a believer in Christ Jesus. For it felt like He was chasing my heart. In my most vulnerable moments, my trust needed to lie somewhere other than myself. I am very good at taking care of myself, thank you very much. Suddenly my life takes a turn, and I better get ready for the unchartered course it will take. One day at a time. We all have a story within us. This shall be my story.

CONTENTS

CHAPTER ONE

GETTING TO KNOW ME

MY PERSONAL BIOGRAPHY

I was born in 1959 when the cost of a gallon of gas was 25 cents. The average cost of a new house was $12,400, a new car $2,200, movie tickets were $1.00, and a loaf of bread 20 cents! It was also the year when Alaska became the forty-ninth and Hawaii the fiftieth state of the United States. Michael was the most popular baby boy name and Mary was for baby girls. The first Barbie doll was launched by Mattel and I became the third of six children weighing in at almost ten pounds. So aside from Fidel Castro becoming a communist prime minister for Cuba, 1959 was a decent year! I enjoyed reading about these fun facts of '59.

I have two sisters and three brothers. I was raised in a traditional home with traditional values. My ethnicity is part English, French, and Mexican. I wouldn't say I have fair skin, but medium skin tone. Both my parents were Catholic and we were raised in this faith. We lived on the tropical island of beautiful San Juan, Puerto Rico, for almost six years. There I learned to swim just beyond the breakers in the ocean by the age of four. I loved it! From the moment my father put me in the water, I felt like a fish.

Otherwise, sunny California was our home. I was an above-average student, enjoyed athletics, was very competitive, relentless, and not just in sports. I played tennis as a youth, water skied, snow skied, but swimming has always been my favorite sport. I swam competitively on the local swim teams, and then in high school. I competed for almost twelve years, and many of those years we trained twice daily in outdoor pools. Early morning and afternoons, with swim meets almost every weekend. When I wasn't swimming, I was either on the tennis court or watching one of my siblings' outdoor sports. We were active kids and our parents were very busy with all six of us heading off here or there. All this outdoor activity was without sunblock. If my mother knew of sunscreen, I am sure it was not in the budget for applying it on six children every single day several times a day, while outside in our bathing suits. Putting a T-shirt on when we had enough sun was our sunscreen. I do recall zinc-oxide. You know, that popular skin protection paste that had been around forever. I can only recall my father slathering this white paste all over his nose and lips whenever we were outside. This was never an attractive look on him, but especially not on a girl. Let alone a teenager.

But it was all about the tan when I was a teenager, and I always had a head start. My sport being an outdoor sport and, as a bonus, I was in a bathing suit! As I got older, swim workouts were longer and twice daily. Meets occupied our every weekend. Give me the baby oil, Crisco, cocoa-butter or whatever greasy thing I can put on my skin to help this tan along! I know there are some of you reading this right now who know exactly what I mean. Then as a young mom, I had no time to just lie in the sun. So I did the next best thing: lay in tanning bed for the quicker tan. Even when tanning beds came out, they claimed it was safer than the sun's UV rays. What a great invention, and it only took fifteen to twenty minutes per session! I did not know all of these contributing factors, in the detail of risk, associated to skin cancer as I do now. **But, if you can relate to this, make an appointment with your dermatologist if you have not done so before**. Being proactive in this area may save your life. When you read the risks associated with melanoma skin cancer, it looks like I set myself up for this and I did, but I didn't even know I was doing it. Now, I need to be smarter about tackling the challenge before me. It will be crucial.

I married my high-school sweetheart in 1979, and graduated from a registered nurse program in 1980. We had grown our family with the addition of two daughters by 1984. I worked on the pre- and postsurgical floor and practiced my newfound skills in our local hospital until 1986. Wanting more of an eight-to-five job and to avoid the weekend shifts with hospital nursing to enjoy motherhood, I went to work for my OB-GYN as the in-office nurse. I enjoyed my experience in this specialty, so I decided to go back to school to further my career options. I attended San Jose State University, School of Nursing, continuation program, for my family nurse practitioner license in 1989. Once that was completed, I would continue in the program to obtain my specialty in obstetrics and gynecology soon after. Within the couple of years that followed, I completed a certificate program in reproductive endocrinology and infertility and obtained a level 1 ultra-sonography certificate. Our practice had a very strong infertility program that I prided myself in being a part of. We had much success in helping women conceive.

I worked in private practice for almost twenty-plus years with two of the finest, respected, and most knowledgeable physicians in town. Both of them took pride in staying current, and had excellent work ethic. I learned so much from both of them throughout the years. The experience was an education in itself and allowed me to build a broader knowledge base. This was the foundation I needed and would take with me as I worked part-time and became the GYN or women's health specialist in the student health center at a state university only twenty minutes from my home.

My time at the college health center was priceless. I found the seven years I spent in this role to be extremely rewarding. I enjoyed my coworkers, which made it pleasant to go to work. Aside from the clinical appointments like complete physical exams, pap smears, STD testing, birth control, and other routine female issues, I found I gradually morphed into the role of a counselor as I began to see its need. The college years for some may bring the most difficult of growing pains. It can be the 'Year of Firsts'—first relationship, first breakup, first sexual experience, first sexual violation, first sexually transmitted disease, or even a pregnancy and maybe abortion. Then there is the first time away from home, the first failed class, the first time intoxicated, first time without friends, and the loneliness associated with that. Nowadays with the social-media world, it can destroy a person in the time it takes to tweet something. The anxiety, depression, and eating disorders during these college years can occur more frequent than most people think.

During my time at the college as the GYN practitioner, I felt there might be a need to expose and inform students of these 'growing pains' through the four years on campus. So I considered writing a book about 'All you can expect from college years.' Kind of a guide, awareness, to the reality of all these potential 'firsts,' including the overwhelming emotional lability and its normalcy if it doesn't linger too long. Of course the possible weight gain, but with the end focus goal—of graduation. This book was going to be titled *The Little Pink Book*. The focus was for young women. I was feeling very passionate about this, and even wrote two chapters. I don't know if I will be driven to complete it, as I have been working nonstop, relentlessly driven, and much more passionate to complete this book.

As for my writing skills, the scope of my writing talents are minimal. I wrote and developed some of the policies and protocols for our private office. I did some educational in-service handouts in this setting, as well as wrote some medical language text for our electronic medical records system. My husband and I renewed our marriage vows and we wrote our vows—this counts, right? We celebrated our thirty-sixth wedding anniversary in Maui in September 2015, with our youngest daughter and her family in attendance. A priceless moment.

Then the past year was the year of the 'Birthday Poem/Prayer,' in which I wrote a poem/prayer for each member of my immediate family; husband, daughters and their husbands, each grandchild, and gave it to them on their birthday. I did not do this because of my diagnosis; this was a thought prior to even knowing I would have cancer. It was only after my son-in-law insisted on "no gifts' for his birthday in February. So I thought, *What else can I do so he knows how much I really love him and am thankful for him being a part of our lives?* The poem/prayer is what I came up with. After I read a couple of different poem/prayers I had written to my mother, she said to me, "I want a prayer," so I wrote one for her and gave it to her on Mother's Day. Which led to writing one for my sisters also. I have one left to do and that is for my youngest grandson, Easton. He just turned one, but I wanted to get to know his personality a little more before I write his poem/prayer.

I have included the prayer to my mother below. She loved it.

Mother's Day Prayer

God knew when He made mothers
How important they would be
So He made them strong, with hearts of Gold
And You made her ~ just for me

You blessed her with six children
Three girls and three strong boys
And she never seem to tire
With sleepless nights, through all the noise

There were countless baths and stories
Many kisses, hugs and smiles
Then swim meets, games, and matches
She chauffeured us miles and miles

The years have passed and we've all grown
The memories we'll hold dear
Her job is done, it is our job now
To love her through the years

Please bless my precious mother
Whose heart You made of Gold
You made her in Your Image
Now make me in her mold

Happy Mother's Day ~ Lita '17

Through my years as a midlevel provider, I experienced a spectrum of diagnoses in my area of expertise. There were the 'good news' moments with joy, success, and cure. But in the area of medicine no matter the specialty, there will be moments we witness overwhelming pain and the devastating, always unwelcomed news of death. The shoe is on the other foot now. I am the patient and not the provider, which is a very uncomfortable and humbling place for me. All of this I have just shared with you does not qualify me as an expert in skin cancer. My personal history is—I have experienced all three—squamous cell carcinoma, basal cell carcinoma, and malignant melanoma. Oh, no, I don't pretend to be an expert. I am very thankful I had excellent physicians to guide me through this trek, as it did have its rugged patches. But I would learn about it along the way.

I want to preface this all by saying I by no means think my news is the most devastating news, nor the 'worst of the worst' that one can receive. I truly recognize this. But I had reason for worry and concern. I have known many people who have had to endure a more difficult path to wellness. For some, no recovery at all was in their future. Some of you reading this right now may have been dealt a much more difficult and trying diagnosis in life. My hope is that you find the daily courage and strength you need to continue tackling your own challenges, cancer or not. How do you chose to replenish your strength as the daily grind can become so fatiguing, frightening, and all-consuming? Because it does take courage and strength while in the battle. A battle where fear and loneliness can creep in and surround you. Sometimes the biggest battle fought isn't the cancer, or an illness, but the emotional battle we suddenly find ourselves in. We are not prepared for this emotional turmoil or how to deal with it. How do you get by?

There are those who have suffered intense and devastating issues with poor prognosis, even worse treatment options and risks. Having to succumb to an illness is a very real part of life. It is the sign our time here on this earth, or our journey, will come to a close. Most of us are unprepared, and we may never feel ready for it all to end. But no matter how we choose to tackle our illness, most of the time it is with the hope to be cured or, at minimum, extend our life span. For this world is all we know, and we do not want to exit it any sooner than is necessary. I have the Hope of Eternal Life as I walk on my journey toward heaven. To experience and know what this Hope is—is my prayer for all humanity.

MY CHRISTIAN BIOGRAPHY

I was raised with a Catholic upbringing. I feel compelled to share some of my Christian background because I think there is something to be said about why this current trek has a spiritual hold on me. I was introduced to God at young age. I began going to church as early as I can remember. The 'basic' foundation was laid and I have carried this faith with me, and hope to continue this walk until my death. Maybe death will seem less frightening—I don't know. But no matter what age we are when we first get that exposure to church and God, with some of us it just means we have more years under our belt. It may not mean we have been in a relationship with Him for long, like myself. A relationship with God is different from just believing in Him. My early introduction to God may be the reason during this challenge I have felt a 'pull.' But the very slow transition I made from being a 'believer' to being a 'believer in a relationship' with my Creator is the joy to life itself. Both are Heaven-bound, but I gratefully welcomed what had evolved.

Now I, as we all, can experience the irritability in life's demands, with family or duties. I am not perfect and I write this with my trials, complaints, and frustrations throughout. One can have faith, one can even exude joy and still live in the reality of frustrations and pain. But the good that can come from a spiritual pull can manifest itself in other areas of our life and with each other. If we were perfect, then without fail others would feel the love, encouragement, hope, goodness, compassion, empathy, and the giving selflessly all of the time. Oh, that's Heaven, and I still remain human—on this earth—with you.

Can people be this way without knowing God? After all, there are 'good' people in this world, both those who are believers and those who do not believe in God. What and who qualifies as 'good'? Is just being a 'good' person, versus an evil person, good enough in God's eyes? And what about the people who say they are a Christian but whose hypocrisy or pretense is clearly visible. Then there are your Sunday Christians and that is all. How and does all this matter to God? And if so, how will we be judged? That is, if this judgement matters at all to us. As I am recovering from my previous surgery, these are but a few of the questions I would become curious about. How deep is my faith and His mercy now? What are His rules?

Now I have never experienced an AH-HA moment like some believers have. My Christian faith has continued to evolve over the years. Some years have been more inclusive of Christ Jesus than others. But there was never an AH-HA moment. I don't think there needs to be either. The reality of that AH-HA moment may simply be the ongoing comfort and joy we experience in the depths of our soul knowing that we will be welcomed into the Kingdom of Heaven. It is a daily spiritual sustenance of goodness.

I was around six or seven years old living in Puerto Rico when my very first religious memory occurred. I can vividly recall one Good Friday, my parents taking us to a reenactment of the Stations of the Cross. It is a Catholic devotion that commemorates Jesus Christ's last day on Earth as man through a series of fourteen images. It is also called the Way of Sorrow or Via Crucis. The only station I remember specifically was the Station of the Crucifixion (Jesus dies on the cross). I can remember it was in the early afternoon; we stood at the bottom of a small hill and I was looking up. We could not see what was on the other side. I must have been four feet tall or so back then. I remember seeing the first full-size cross being raised by ropes, very slowly. Then the second cross was slowly raised, and there were men on them, bound with ropes. Then they raised the third and center cross where Jesus would be hanging, and there was also a man on this cross. His arms outstretched and he had what appeared to be like a crown of thorns on his head. He had a bloodstained face and side, with a white drape around his pelvis. The cross seemed to loom over the other two and appeared so big. I am sure there must have been gasps from the crowd; it was frightfully impressive. Suddenly it fell darker and there were sound effects, like the roaring of thunder and clashing, like the boom of lightning. I don't remember how I felt. Fear, sadness, even sorrow I suppose ... I was young. Needless to say, it left an impression. This vivid memory has been with me all these years only to resurface now as I began writing my Christian bio. I shared this memory with my mother last week and she recalled the impressive theatrical display, as did my older brother who was probably nine or ten at the time. He said it was one of the scariest things he had ever seen. Can you even imagine witnessing the crucifixion in real time? What kind of impression would that have left? Would it have made believing in Jesus easier?

We as a family would attend church on a Sunday morning. I admit at times it felt more like an obligation or even a chore to attend. But I liked wearing a dress, and even on vacation, even if we were only camping, I made sure I had my dress and nylons. Remember nylons? No one wears them anymore! I would make sure I had my proper attire to attend church wherever we were, and I got kidded about it. Even to this day, my siblings remember this and laugh at me. So I was exposed to church and God at a young age and now with some life situations behind me, my faith has evolved into something more. But I don't remember when I became 'more serious' about my faith. Most of the time when I did attend church, I was always glad I had made the effort to go. I think I was around age thirty-five or so when I let 'it' become more important to me—or I took 'it' more seriously. But once I did, I began to feel a change in my soul.

I was sort of the middle child—but without issues. I had three brothers and two sisters and we all played together a lot. I for some reason loved to play school. I confess that I stole the missalettes from the pews in church at the age of nine, so I could have some reading material for my students when we would play 'school' in my garage. I used to recruit neighbor kids and some of my siblings to be the students. I became a thief and a teacher at age nine! My sisters remember this and they were my most difficult and unruly students.

My siblings and I all attended parochial school. We had the uniforms and cute little caps, and we had a special uniform for Fridays. I went to Catholic school up through the seventh grade. I received some of the Sacraments; Baptism, First Communion or Eucharist, Confirmation, and Marriage. My husband converted to Catholicism two months before we were to be married. We did marriage counseling that was required before we were to wed, and the priest had said we were testing at opposing ends of the spectrum. We were oil and water. I say the old saying may be true—opposites do attract! I was certainly the more extroverted and social one and he was more introverted, athletic, and handsome. I needed to be around people to reenergize and he would prefer to be alone to reenergize.

My husband learned more about Catholicism in just two months of study than I did in nineteen years. We eventually married in the Catholic Church. Married by that same priest who took us through our marriage counseling. I think he liked both of us very much. We were both barely twenty years old. Since I have been a believer as far back as I can remember, I don't remember ever doubting that God was real. But I saw my husband striving for a relationship with Our Lord, where I was recognizing myself to be just a 'believer.' It was after the baptism of our first daughter when we knew we wanted to change our church affiliation for this exact reason. He wanted to learn how to have a relationship with our God and I would still be a believer. But we were committed to attending church as a family and not split up. So we began attending a Protestant church and we raised our daughters with an introduction to Christ in the Protestant church at a very young age.

I did some volunteering here and there for Sunday school or other activities along the way. I listened to sermons, some better than others. I have never read the Bible in its entirety. But when I do start reading the written word, I am enthralled and admit at times confused. Off and on through the years I would read daily devotionals and spend time reading, pondering. This was never a daily routine for me. It was important and it was not important. Still just a believer. Never took notes. I am not sure why this has 'stuck.' I am not an expert in the Bible, again no pretense. We still attend the Protestant church and are hit and misses with Sunday services. Some reasons are simply lame: too tired, entertained last night, have company visiting. I feel bad that He doesn't get the front seat all of the time. I apologize for the neglect. I am a sinner. I will always look forward to our next visit. I am never disappointed when I do attend church and always manage to feel lifted and reenergized to begin a new week. It is food for my soul and how I appreciate this now.

As I mentioned there were certain memories that came to surface as I explore with my writing. I have experienced several visions or dreams that have come to me in the middle of the night over the years. They are always, always, in the middle of the night. You need not be convinced this really happened or believe me, as it is my good fortune. Most of the visions or glimpses had comforted me. But not all of my visions were comforting: two of them have been very dark, but I will only share one with you. As you read through this, you will find other visions included here and there. But the very first vision I ever remember having was when I was twenty-seven years old and about fourteen weeks pregnant with my third child. It was early April. I had a fever of 103, my neck was causing me excruciating pain, and I was on antibiotics. I had not felt the baby move as yet. It was the middle of the night that I recall a dark vision and a visit from several dark-hooded and cloaked spirits, all with sickles. The gang of them glided into my room as if floating, and they were all peering down at me, surrounding me. I felt like they wanted my baby. In my sleep I said, "Go away. You can't have my baby." I immediately woke up, drenched in sweat. Maybe this was a fever breaking? Hallucinating, I don't know. I don't need to know, because I remember this so vividly. I have never had a visit from them since, yet I have had fevers with other illnesses since.

When I mentioned this dream to my doctor at my next appointment, he said that some women have complained of this type of 'dark dream' experience before. I was worried that something must be wrong. When we did the Doppler test to find the heartbeat, he couldn't pick it up. So we proceeded to the in-office ultrasound. I of course knew what to look for right away. I saw plenty of amniotic fluid, a perfectly formed fetus with all its organs. It had both hands and I even counted five fingers on one of its hands. The hand was very still but was completely open, like a wave of a hand. I saw the head, body, two legs, everything was there, except … the heartbeat. I said to the doctor, "You don't see a heartbeat either, do you?" Sure enough there was no heartbeat. I was fourteen weeks pregnant. The measurements had shown the baby was only shy of twelve weeks. Which meant it had passed earlier in the week before. I think the cloaked spirits were there to collect. Then the options were reviewed with me and I had chosen to have a procedure done the following day. Then I grieved the loss of my baby.

My husband didn't really seem to get too emotional or grieve. It had not become real to him as yet. He had not felt a connection, and he is a great father. But he could manage to comfort me. I am a firm believer—mothers do not forget specifics. I do remember thinking, *If I hear "It's Mother*

Nature's way" one more time.... This comment does not help. I tried so hard not to say this in my practice, but sometimes I would slip. This is also one of those life's 'why' questions that has NO answer.

It was almost two years after this miscarriage when my second vision came to me. Again, it was the middle of the night. I heard beautiful music and saw a meadow so rich in color palettes of blossoms everywhere. I specifically remember this dream took place close to what my due date would have been, in October sometime. There were little children, boys and girls happy and laughing, and all were dressed in white gowns. They were playing and dancing about within this low picket wooded fence area. They couldn't go beyond the fence. I did not see any adults with them. Then suddenly a little blonde child maybe two years old stepped up on the bottom rung of the fence and started to wave at me. She had a page-boy haircut and a white gown that stopped right above her ankles. She had no shoes on. She was beautiful and she knew me! How can this be? I woke my husband up in the early hours of the morning to tell him, "We have a baby girl, and she is waiting for us in Heaven." Then I described my vision to him. I was comforted. He, my Lord, had comforted me by giving me a glimpse into Heaven to see our baby girl. I often thought of this vision as my reward for shooing off the black-hooded cloaked spirits just two years before.

Our baby would have been due in October of 1987 and I miscarried in April of 1987, so this vision came to me in October 1989. Two years later and I don't know why. Maybe so I could see her precious face. For those of you who have seen the movie, *The Shack*, do you recall the part in the movie when the Holy Spirit allowed the father to finally see his daughter because he missed her so much and felt so guilty? How she was playing in the beautiful meadow with all the other little children. I watched this movie alone when my husband was traveling. When I saw that scene, I choked up and my eyes filled with tears. I recalled how the Lord blessed me with the glimpse of her, waiting, joyfully, happily in Heaven, in the meadow. Rent this movie and watch it with a box of Kleenex! I am not going to spoil it. It falls under the genre "Realistic Fiction." You can take away whatever you want from it; what He reveals is up to you to consider as possible.

God does know my heart even when I am not visiting with Him. He knows your heart too. Even with all your questions. He knows I am a sinner, and that I am human. He knows all, and does not need to be made aware of anything. He is my instant, my constant, and my 'Go To.' He is in everything, everywhere, and in every moment. I know God wants to be my center.

CHOSEN RESOURCES TO FUEL MY STRENGTH

I've already divulged that I am not a Bible-versed follower. I don't have scripture memorized like some may. I do believe in the Bible. I miss church on occasion. Which I am not proud of admitting. I am a Christian and I love the Lord, but I am definitely not claiming to be an expert in theology. I do feel that God knows what I am about, and possibly that most people who have met me would say I am a 'good person.' During my recovery, I did however experience growth with the maturing of my faith during my recent trek. By maturing of my faith, I mean I reeducated myself and tried to explore and understand the history of the Bible, read Scripture and understand the Trinity. I 'started' spending time in readings and pondering these avenues I chose to gain my encouragement from. Then began my scriptural journaling on what touched me, or became pertinent to me. I tried to tie whatever emotion I was struggling with during each challenge with my cancer and see what scripture had to say about it. I found I used my Bible resource as the 'dictionary' for tackling emotions, which were intense and unfamiliar to me. What does the Bible say about it? I soon discovered this was not an ordinary dictionary, and as I explored more, this dictionary would prove to be nourishing, inspiring, encouraging, and validating. Even with my baby steps, it would grant me grace and then strengthened my Hope as the challenge for healing progressed.

I also would engage in a mixture of readings and online sermons. The sermons were from Charles Stanley, a senior pastor at a First Baptist Church in Georgia and the founder and president of In Touch Ministries. Many scriptures from the NIV *Bible*, and also *The Life Principles Bible* by Charles F. Stanley. It is the NIV bible with which he provides additional life lessons pertinent to the scripture for a better understanding in the early days. He makes things very clear as to what a particular verse may be conveying, and he incorporates the life lessons for this world of here and now. I would also read from a daily devotional, *Jesus Calling*, written by Sarah J. Young who shared she has had melanoma on two occasions. She does not elaborate to what extent on this at all, just gives a mention to it. Every day her devotionals were inspiring, as if God were speaking directly to me. I would read her devotional and then look up the scripture verses she had drawn her inspiration from. There were so many occasions when I would be feeling a particular way and I opened up either the bible or a devotional and it addressed the emotion so perfectly and provided encouragement for me. Time after time this occurred, and that alone spoke volumes to me, as if the Holy Spirit were seated right in front of me having a conversation. I am sure now He was. I could not believe how 'perfectly pertinent' so many messages in another daily devotional I would read, called *Women's Daily Devotional*, were. These are devotionals written by many different women who have enjoyed both the joys and the struggles of Christian living, and were willing to share their experiences in triumphs or trials with us. Familiar names to you.

Then there was a book recommended to my husband called *The Strength You Need*, written brilliantly by Pastor Robert J. Morgan, who is the bestselling author of *Then Sings My Soul* and *The Red Sea Rules*. Both of which I am looking forward to reading.

The Strength You Need is a book that offers encouragement and strength when you feel like there is nothing left in you. You are physically, mentally, and spiritually depleted and drained. You can be exhausted just with life itself and all your duties within it. You certainly do not have to be stricken with an illness to read it. The author has chosen what he considers to be the twelve great strength passages of the Bible. He expands on these scripture verses with personal stories as well as makes some parallels for us to see the strength the Lord imparts as depicted in biblical stories. His wife who has challenges of her own adds her personal experience at the end of each chapter pertinent to the topic of the chapter. Very sweet idea, and this makes it real. Very here and now. I became inspired and passionate in the variety of readings I was engaged in almost daily, and sometimes for hours. Such a great gift to me. Thank you Pastor Robert J. Morgan and all the rest of the authors that inspired me. It is a must read if you need to find your strength, or simply find encouragement in replenishing it.

Last, I read the book *The Language of God* by Dr. Francis S. Collins, a scientist who presents evidence for belief. This book may be a challenging read, but only because it is written by a highly qualified and brilliant scientist/geneticist. In a nutshell, it is during his assignment as head of the Human Genome project that took over a decade to map out when his journey unfolds. He went from being an atheistic scientist to a scientist who says ten years later when the project is complete, "It's a happy day for the world. It is humbling for me and awe-inspiring to realize that we have caught the first glimpse of our own instruction book, previously known 'only' to God." His work is with DNA, 'the hereditary code of life' through building of a human being. He makes his stunning case through modern science for God and for science. He can refute every argument against faith by scientists, as well as support some scientific truths for religious skeptics. He discovers the beauty of how science and Christianity are complementary, and sights how they "reinforce each other's existence."

Reminder: scripture for the NIV Bible quoted will be *italicized*. I would recommend checking these sources out, as they all provided and imparted wisdom and encouragement when I had felt empty. All my sources helped me stay focused on the bigger picture, finding *Strength* and ultimate *Peace* in my journey.

With regards to skin cancer awareness portion of this book, I have included educational information that I pooled from multiple resources. Some definitions are just that: they don't change, just the verbiage in describing them does. **This is a little more informative than basic understanding, but is not to take the place of anything your personal dermatologist tells you.** Yet it is more comprehensive in other areas that I had a personal journey/experience in. You may be less enthused about reading some of it, but you can refer to it whenever. Some forms of literature I received was from Stanford Cancer Research or from my team of physicians at Stanford during this process. Other information was researched through the American Cancer Society (ACS), *Journal of the American Academy of Dermatology*

(JAAD), National Cancer Institute (NCI) with regards to skin cancer. NCI has the accurate, up-to-date, comprehensive cancer information from the US government's principal agency for cancer research, and it also recognizes Stanford Dermatology as a major contributor to the advancement of skin cancer research. And last the Skin Cancer Foundation (SCF). You can find many of these sources online. Again, you will find any references made to skin cancer in **black bold print**.

I have never been a big reader. There is always so much reading involved in staying current with all the changes or new studies in medicine that I rarely had time for reading something for leisure. Maybe because this diagnosis was a hefty health scare or life event, I decided to reach for something that may provide encouragement or give me fuel. Something to help me understand when there is nothing else I can do. People tried so hard to be encouraging and say the right thing when I would share what I was going through, but some just don't know how to respond. Maybe because they didn't understand the gravity, others just stumble. Both are understandable and that is okay. It is hard to know what to say other than 'I'm sorry.' So I would slowly begin reading scripture in March of 2017, but more regularly than I ever did before. I had just received news that was unchartered in my life's book. I had many diagnostic tests scheduled ahead of me to determine how extensive or progressive the cancer was. So I had a heightened sense of fear and worry, in which I had never experienced this intensity either. Does anyone really enjoy being the patient? I am so humbled.

In the beginning, after the second diagnosis of malignant melanoma was made and waiting seemed like all I was doing, I experienced many days that were 'sprinkled' with fear, anxiety, loneliness, and just frustration with my body. The diagnosis of cancer was very real. It was a shock. The courage it takes to tackle cancer I had never thought about before, and now it is here and needs my attention. I would also not realize nor understand the strength my God could and would provide me, because I had never given Him the chance before. I-had-never-given-Him-the-chance-before. I just heard how that sounded. I do so many things unassisted and I am very 'capable.' Which is a word I prefer using instead of 'controlling.' But to not give Him a chance to do with me what He will? What will be in store for me if I would only let Him—mold me like clay to a Potter, be the Captain of my vessel, or the Painter of my canvas?

SCRIPTUAL JOURNALING BEGINS

For some reason one morning, I decided to listen to my very first online sermon with Pastor Charles Stanley, founder of In-Touch Ministries. On that particular morning and this particular sermon, he had been insistent on note taking. I thought, *Surely he's not talking to me.* Then he literally stopped preaching and said he wanted to see more people taking notes, for them to get their pens and paper out. It was almost like he saw me just sitting all quiet on my couch sipping on my coffee and he was looking right at me. Yikes, so I hit the pause button, got up off the couch, picked up a legal pad and pen, restarted his sermon, and began taking notes. I thought, *Why not. Really, I'm not going anywhere anytime soon. There is a first time for everything.* I can look back and reread this richness anytime I feel like it. This first online sermon moment became the little seed that began my writing and I didn't even know it. Nor did I know where this discovery would lead me, unless I tried.

It would take months before I would be overwhelmingly compelled to put it all together in this format, to share with anyone who would be interested, at a later date. I do not know how it will be received, nor in which avenues it will be accessible to read. I am just going to continue with my writing. But this will be twofold, with my attention to detail in both my medical and spiritual journey. So walk with me.

If you have ever wondered, 'What if God is real,' I hope you can keep an open mind as you read the spiritual journey I embraced. I absolutely know that my walk of faith will not be your walk of faith. We all have to choose our own path in our own time while here on earth. It may have God in it, but for some it may not. If you are curious, my sincere hope when you read this is that it leaves you at a minimum wanting to ask one more question about what it means to know God. For His Grace is precious, His Mercy is exhaustive, and to trust in the Hope for Eternal Life by allowing Him to simply 'love you' is free for you to discover. The foundation for me was poured long ago; now I absolutely cannot ignore this pull, so I will continue to be led and I will continue to write.

My spiritual journey was first and foremost in my desire to put this down on paper. But my medical background had created an additional tug in the area of skin cancer awareness. I wanted to include my personal journey, with all my frustrations through the challenges of this cancer, as well as help broaden the awareness to include a knowledge base regarding the number one reported and diagnosed cancer for as many people as possible. Again, this area of writing for me was prompted as I advanced through the different phases of procedures or challenges for this type of cancer, while aiding myself for the best possible outcome. Survival. What a variety of knowledgeable team members I had in this with me.

If you are in medicine, a provider, or anyone who has direct contact with a cancer patient, I hope as long as you are in the role, you thirst to increase your knowledge base. The confidence exuding from such a broad knowledge base as you educate your patient aids in establishing a trust-based relationship. This relationship provides a comfort to us, with a trust in you. We patients need a confident and well-informed clinician to guide us through this trek. We stay hopeful as we trust we are getting the best and most current information to make a well-informed decision for the challenges ahead. Our ignorance in this unchartered territory yields to fear within us. No matter the significance, you will witness the degree of impact this type of news can have on a patient, as it did me and my family. The ripple effect, so to speak. The reality is the "C" word, cancer, starts an entire sequence of events within oneself and a family. Which is what I have tried to capture in this book. Patients need to sense the empathy and confidence by you, as we feel you are in this with us. The fact of the matter is cancer is real, bad news does happen, and it has to be delivered. We are counting on you to bring your 'BEST' every time. Don't let me become- just another cancer patient.

I like counting on myself and making my own decisions. But these become tougher when I don't feel well informed or don't completely understand the particulars. I needed and wanted opinions, direction, and guidance. I was very direct with some of my physicians with questions like, "What would you do, if you were me?" Or "If I was your sister, what would your advice be?" "Did I understand these risks correctly?" My team was excellent in providing me with answers, but of course the decisions are always the patients'. The decisions had to be mine. My post-op trial will definitely be an education that my physicians will recall for any future patients who may experience the same thing. It may have seemed outside the normal course, but for me as the patient, I still consider it a varying degree of 'normal' post-op recovery course. Maybe just at the upper end. A setback will require the need for patience in my recovery, which is proven here. A tolerance for pain and patience is needed in most recoveries and it's the one thing we are the worst at. Well, I am anyway. There were many blogs regarding post-op courses for sentinel lymph node dissections of the axilla, but fewer detailed ones for complete axillary dissections and what limitations may await, another reason I felt compelled to write my experience down and expand on the breadth of symptoms that befell me, but tried to make it even more informative, so I include what burdened me.

As I began interacting with friends and family, unveiling some of my current challenges of my health issue, it became evident that many people did not know what malignant melanoma was, let alone how serious it could be if left untreated. And if they had heard of skin cancer, they certainly were not aware of the different types nor the risks associated with these cancers if left untreated. So many people are still very unaware of the effects of skin cancer.

Medical Pearl

Bottom line, as with any potential life-threatening illness, the earlier it is identified, the sooner proper treatment can begin. Sometimes early detection is the life-saving key element. Never ignore a change in a skin lesion, or a new lesion.

It was after my second diagnosis in February 2017, when I was shopping, that I purchased a pink journal at a local little shop and on the cover it read, 'Think Happy, Be Happy.' So I bought it, only because it was really cute, and set it down on our coffee table. It sat there for a couple of months. Then one day in April, a Sunday to be exact, I just picked it up and started writing my emotional experience down. I would add a thought down here and there, as my journey unfolded. My scriptural note taking was on a legal pad and had begun a month or so prior. My notes were from sources of the moment I would read, and they varied daily. Random choices, from scripture verses to daily devotionals, etc. as I mentioned before. I could refer to these notes and reread them with the hope they would provide me courage and strength in my days ahead.

It would be safe to say my writing began when my emotions were so raw, fragile, and surfaced that you could almost touch them. Surely I was wearing 'worry' on my sleeve. Writing was very therapeutic: it kept evolving and seemed to come to me easily. It was my release, especially trying to keep a brave front. Only after I would share some of my notes with family would they have a mere glimpse of my worry. I think this was unnerving for some. I truly began to realize, and believed even with all the fearful moments that would come and go, that I was never alone. I was already enjoying my choices for my spiritual hour, or two or three. The truth behind anxious moments and fear, coupled with loneliness, feels overwhelming and may become paralyzing. The loneliness I would feel was simply because I felt I could not share my innermost concerns or thoughts with anyone. Not that I felt unloved or unworthy, but I think because I am a social person and all the alone time I had on my hands contributed to this feeling. It also felt too burdensome to share. I think I am viewed as a strong woman, and I needed to stay strong for the entire family to be able to get through this without their lives falling apart at work or at home. I have amazingly strong daughters. But this type of news when everyone is already wondering how all this is going to end can create an entirely new daily worry.

The only time I fell apart (burst into tears for a few minutes) was when my husband's brother, Tom, came for a short visit and I shared how frightened I was. I had shared I had an 80 percent survival rate in five years. I cried in his embrace, with my mother-in-law in the room. I wept for several minutes and told him I have not fallen apart in front of Scott, my husband,

and nor would I. My fear and loneliness slowly over time, several months even, transformed and morphed into 'Power' and 'Peace.' I felt the rawness of a multitude of emotions during this challenge, but these two had their grip on me. What I felt as my weakness was being carried, lifted, I cannot explain it, but 'Power and Peace' would make their presence known with a visit here and there, a burden lifted when I needed it most.

So this pink journal of mine, *Think Happy, Be Happy*, was meant to become my *Little Pink Book*. The book that I have not completed as of yet. Is the fact that it is pink a coincidence? This pink journal is leading me down this writing path instead. I perceive this redirection is from the power of the Holy Spirit. But hey, that's me. Maybe after this I will be so moved to complete the 'other' *Little Pink Book*.

This is simply my personal experience, my opinions, my views with these events simultaneously affecting me. In regards to my spiritual revival, it is my story. It is my testimony so to speak, and how I chose to cope through the fear with this initial news of cancer for my spiritual wellness. The treatments and choices I would make to tackle this, with an unknown recovery regarding limitations, is awaiting me. The mental and physical challenge it presented was not only to me but to my family also. Most importantly, how I felt the presence of the Holy Spirit through it all. I felt the comfort in knowing I was never really alone, but then shared in a moment when I KNEW I was not alone. As I began journaling through this recent challenge, I began to recall and expose past spiritual memories that I had not thought about for quite some time. These collective memories have unveiled spiritual clarity and permanency for my life. I believe each had a hold from within, and must have been my sustenance through the years as a believer and now it has evolved into my story on paper. The bonus was now finding I was in a relationship with my Creator, and the exact moment I would and could recognize this. My hope is that it may make you ponder a little longer and question a little more if there is something to this Heavenly Father. I have never doubted but I am human, and I have experienced the fear that goes hand in hand with a cancer diagnosis. Being consumed with fear is an unhealthy distraction. It was through this recent medical challenge that I would discover just how powerful of a life-changing grip it 'all' would have on me.

Lastly, as you turn the pages please know this was written from my heart. At times it may read as complaints or what you may think are insignificant consequences to a surgical intervention. But I wanted to share 'everything' I was experiencing. I know some of you will relate to what I have experienced, and I recognize that some of you have suffered so much more than I can even imagine. Even those of you who have had or will choose the same surgical path, our outcomes may not be similar, but the experience will certainly be identifiable. One thing we will share is the reality the difficulties a single day may pose, because we lived it—to different extents. Sharing my family life's moments and it's frailty with you as they occur in real time causes me to pause, be thankful, and appreciate all that should be truly important to me.

CHAPTER TWO

SKIN CANCER
AWARENESS BEGINS

MY FIRST DERMATOLOGY VISIT-
THE DISCOVERY

This new skin cancer awareness began for me in November 2013. This is what I meant when I said I stumbled into this cancer institution without knowing all the glowing accolades or even what my relationship with this team of physicians would come to mean to me. I had a friend who wanted to go shopping at Stanford Shopping mall, and she asked me to join her. But first she needed to see her dermatologist, and suggested I make an appointment with her dermatologist for the same day as well. So I did, and there you have it.

She saw me, did a full body skin examination, and spotted the lesion on my upper right post neck area. She recommended and performed a shave biopsy right then. My friend and I went to lunch and shopped. I bought a beautiful huge wrought-iron lantern at Pottery Barn. It is a unique piece and every time I look at it, I can recall the events that unfolded on this day. I received a phone call three days later confirming malignant melanoma stage I. I was referred for a wide reexcision of the lesion within two weeks. It is very important to make sure all the borders are clear, which will minimize the chance for recurrence. I had seen my local dermatologist for a full-body skin check just eight months or so prior, and he did not spot this lesion. This was not a coincidence either, no way.

After the multiple Holy Spirit moments that I encountered throughout this past year, I do not believe in coincidences anymore. It may even change your minds too. This was a gift from the Holy Spirit. While I was so thankful for the outcome I had in 2013, I did not appreciate the significance it carried until I was diagnosed for a second time with melanoma and all it brought with it this year. **Aside from completely preventing skin cancer, early detection with proper treatment is the next best thing.** Now it does make sense that skin cancer would be ranked as the number one diagnosed cancer (excluding melanoma), due to the fact the integumentary system (skin, hair, nails, and exocrine glands) is the largest organ system of the body. Majority of cancers begin with a single epithelial cell that lines the inside as well as the outside of our bodies. It is also the most exposed organ system.

Medical Pearl

One in five Americans will develop skin cancer in the course of their lifetime. Our risk increases with age. Every time we go out in the sun we increase our risk, as sun exposure is the primary cause. With early detection and proper treatment for basal and squamous cell carcinoma, it can carry a cure rate of over 95 percent. But for malignant melanoma, the statistics are a bit scarier. Again early detection can be life-saving for its victims if it's caught before it spreads to other parts of the body. The survival rate is much, much lower with an invasive melanoma, and depends on many 'individual factors' including staging variables. Statistics will vary from sources you read, so listen to your physician's prognosis and survival rate.

Invasive melanoma is the deadliest of skin cancer diagnosis and it is a frightening thought especially as American Cancer Society (ACS) states approximately **less than 1 percent of all skin cancers are invasive melanoma**. Meaning the survival rate drops significantly with this diagnosis.

No, that trip to Stanford dermatology clinic back in November 2013 was preorchestrated by a Higher Power, so that I may be sitting here right now, today, and typing up my tightly woven, twofold story. A big thank-you to my friend, Jamie, for inviting me to go shopping with her.

My goal is that you find this read to be educational and informative. I hope you learn something new about skin cancer: how it starts, recognizing it (at least enough to seek a professional opinion), identifying your own risks and I will review only my treatment options. Knowledge brings action, and anything that may make you more diligent with your own care and follow-up is a success for all. I have included helpful hints if dealing with early stages of lymphedema, as I did, and in which recalling things to avoid will become second nature. I have purposefully included more detail than some may enjoy reading, but it is all a fairly accurate account and true territory to the treatment of malignant melanoma skin cancer and its surgical options with very real potential complications.

Interestingly enough, some of my post-op trials even my physicians had not encountered with other patients before. So this was new territory for them and thus educational experience for all of us. Not every patient will be offered or choose the same course of treatment, nor will their post-op experience be identical. There is a wide variance in what could be considered 'within normal limits.'

I want this to be an encouraging and inspirational read, as there is always hope with recovery. There may not always be healing and cure, but there is always HOPE. Sometimes the most critical thing left to be healed is the heart. So encouragement to stay proactive with your health means physically, mentally, and spiritually. Finding a way to maintain strength in these areas during this challenge is key no matter how you chose to do so. Find your personal coping source for your physical, mental, and spiritual wellness and make it a daily routine.

COMPLETE REEXCISION OF SKIN LESION

The in-office procedure for complete reexcision of the skin lesion, melanoma, went very smoothly in 2013. After many injections around the lesion area, total numbness was achieved. This procedure took almost two-plus hours. I did not know what to expect. I know how long it takes me to do a complete physical and Pap smear, something so many women dread, but I had no idea a resection like this would take this amount of time. This is to be taken seriously: it is melanoma. Since my husband would be my driver home, I asked for something to help me relax, as I knew I would have difficulty lying there for that length of time. I felt every single needle prick, shallow and deep, until the site was completely numb. The surgeon walked in, and I felt comfortable with her immediately. Now I will lie still and quiet while she did what she did best. I was warned all the injections filled with lidocaine and epinephrine might make me feel jittery, which they did. Two hours later, a pressure dressing was placed and home we would travel. A four- to five-inch well-healed scar remains on my upper right neck. One week later, I would hear the pathology indicated all margins were clear: it was malignant melanoma Stage I. Nothing further needed to be done other than skin check follow-ups every three months. Being diligent with my appointments would prove to be important and my saving grace.

Yes, it needs to get done. Yes, we need to be brave and tough it out. And yes, a lesion less than the size of a pencil eraser tip needs a four-to-five-inch scar for margins to be cleared and the skin to be drawn back together seamlessly. It was an early catch. Thank you, Lord. That Thanksgiving as we gave thanks, there were two more things to be grateful for—my friend and my new dermatologist! At first this all felt like a coincidence, a lucky catch. But could I think of it as a coincidence three years later as I embark down another road with melanoma? No. I can hardly allow myself to imagine the 'what if' I hadn't gone shopping in 2013.

This initial diagnosis with melanoma skin cancer in 2013 did not challenge my faith. Yes I said a prayer, but I cannot really remember how I sought the Lord out at that time. I certainly had no inclination or curiosity to pursue more knowledge in the area of my faith. Something now I recognized—He wanted out of me. Now this spiritual revival has ignited a desire to dig deeper and broaden my knowledge base for my faith in this second round of melanoma skin cancer. The ease of having the first lesion reexcised and all margins cleared, made me felt it was done, over. Thank goodness it all worked out. My dermatologist stated I was considered 'High Risk,' so it would be important for me to be diligent with my sunscreen, sun exposure time, and maintain an every-three-month appointment for my skin checks. So I went on with my life as anyone would, and as most people do I suspect. Being much more conscientious than ever before with all she had reviewed. Even the four-to-five-inch incision—while caring for it, redressing it daily while I was healing up—wasn't enough to test my faith. **Early detection in most cases can improve overall outcomes of almost anything, even cancer. Especially before it enters the lymph nodes.**

MY TREK IS UPON ME

I was due for another full-body skin check in November of 2016 and was coming up on my three years of being clear. She had mentioned to me previously that I would have a 20 percent increase risk for recurrence of melanoma within the first three years. Everything was good, a few minor things, and I was so happy that I had passed the mark. My full-body skin check was good. I would always share the news with my family, as it was a relief to everyone. After the first diagnosis, I made each of my daughters get full-body skin checks by their dermatologist, and they continue to get regular checks even now.

Then in January 2017, I started experiencing a pain deep within my left scapular (shoulder blade) area. I could not pinpoint exactly where it was, nor duplicate the pain with a touch. It was deep and caught my attention. The discomfort was for hours and would disappear. But almost daily for about seven to ten days, I would notice it off and on. Neither Tylenol nor Ibuprofen helped ease this discomfort. I had no other symptoms, no short-ness of breath, chest pain, nausea, fever, cough etc. nothing else. Then one day I had an itch on my back and when I went to scratch it, there was a small lump. My husband took a look and noted I had a 'black mole.' I did not have a black mole on my back before, so another appointment was made.

Medical Pearl

The MAJORITY of melanomas arise from a NEW pigmented lesion and not from a preexisting mole. However, one of the first signs of melanoma could be a change in the size, shape, or color of a preexisting mole. If you have been diagnosed with melanoma, have your children checked by a dermatologist also, especially if they have many freckles. Let the physician tell you they are normal. Don't guess.

Again when she saw me, I saw the same look on her face and the concern in her voice as the first time we had met in 2013. She was quietly concerned the lesion was melanoma. So a shave biopsy was done of the lesion right then and there. **A 'shave biopsy' is a procedure in which a skin abnormality and a thin layer of surrounding skin are removed with a small blade for examination under the microscope.** They inject a numbing agent around the suspect lesion site; once the area is numb, they will take a shave of the area with a blade. They dress it with application of Vaseline and Band-Aid, and you are done. The tissue is sent off to pathology.

A few days later, the news of malignant melanoma Stage I was confirmed. I said, "Ok, well I'd like to request the same surgeon who reexcised the first one. She was great and my scar is barely noticeable now." But there was to be a different option thrown in this time, as this was my second malignant melanoma lesion. I had also updated her on new family history, as my father had just passed of malignant melanoma complications. My present history also includes past lesions of both the other skin cancers—basal cell and squamous cell carcinoma. All these risk factors she took into account, as they impacted the direction she felt would need consideration at the minimum for next steps. This is why I am such a patient advocate: if you don't have confidence in your physician, you have the right to seek a new one out. So let us review how skin cancer can begin in the first place.

WHAT IS SKIN CANCER

Skin cancer, like all cancers, is a disorder of 'uncontrolled' cellular growth. One cell decides it is going off to be by itself and grow however and wherever it wants to. All tumors start as a single cell, then they duplicate and some can multiply quickly. Ninety percent of all cancers begin with the same kind of cell, the **epithelial cell,** which cover us both inside and out. These cells make up our skin and line all our organs. This is where it all begins; for one cell to multiply and become a solid tumor, all it needs is just a little time.

It is my mission in this book to educate, as I've been surprised at how many people are not aware of the types or seriousness of skin cancers. They certainly have not heard of melanoma—nor have any idea what it is, or how devastating it can be. Some have dismissed their own diagnosis because the margins have been cleared, so like my first diagnosis … it's done. Taken care of. But are they staying as diligent as I have been? Every -three-month skin checks for the next three years is what I was advised. **There is a twenty percent increase risk in recurrence within the first three years of detection.** And again, early detection is really important. A skilled physician or dermatologist will see abnormalities we don't even notice.

Sun exposure is the primary cause of all skin cancers. Tanning beds contribute to the increase risk also as they have intense UV rays. There are more than 5 million new cases of skin cancer every year. To put that number in perspective for you, it is more than double the amount of ALL other cancers combined. **There are 90,000 new cases of melanoma annually, and every 54 minutes melanoma claims another life.** This statistic alone should make you want to get a full-body skin check by a dermatologist. **Skin cancer is NOT the number one cancer "killer," but it IS the number one most diagnosed, reported, and treated cancers.**

In a nutshell there are three most common types of skin cancer. Carcinoma is another word for cancer. I include where these cells originate within our skin layers.

UNDERSTANDING THE SKIN LAYERS

First, one must understand the layers of the skin or its makeup. There are three main layers of our skin. For the sake of understanding and simplicity, imagine first a piece of apple pie. With the bottom piecrust layer, the apple filling layer, and the top layer of crust. But not a-la-mode. The longer it's baked in the oven—well, you know what happens.

The **epidermis** is like the top layer of piecrust that becomes golden brown while baking. It is made up of 'epithelial cells,' and it is here where the majority of skin cancers start—basal, squamous, and melanoma cancer as our skin becomes golden brown or burned with sun exposure or other UV exposure.

The **dermis** is the filling layer of the pie. It is made up of all the goodies—fruit, connective tissue, blood vessels, sweat glands, nerves, and hair follicles. This is where you DO NOT want the cancer to penetrate in depth.

The **hypodermis/subcutaneous** is the bottom layer of the piecrust, which is the deepest layer of our skin. This is made up of connective tissues and fats. It is also called the subcutaneous layer by dermatologists. This is even more serious when it comes to skin cancer depth and potential ulceration, for most likely it has entered the lymph system.

THREE DIFFERENT TYPES OF SKIN CANCER

There are typically three different types of skin cancer. All have risk factors associated with them. The first two being discussed are basal cell and squamous cell carcinoma. There is hope in eradicating these skin cancers if caught early enough, where no further action will be required other than to excise it. So it becomes important, if you find yourself in one of the risk categories, to make an appointment and get examined by an experienced dermatologist. Not all primary care physicians know exactly what they are looking at in regards to a skin lesion, so it is okay to ask for a referral to a dermatologist for this. This is why providers need to pay attention to skin lesions when doing annual exams and refer accordingly. When in doubt, check it out!

Basal cell carcinoma (BCC): a skin cancer that begins in the basal cells. These cells line the deepest layer of the epidermis (the outermost layer of the skin, or the underside of the top layer of piecrust sitting closest to the fruit). These cells constantly divide to replace cells lost to wear and tear. The face is the usual area of occurrence. But 80 percent of these lesions will usually appear on the parts of the body that gets a lot of sun exposure. **BCC is the most common form of skin cancer and accounts for the majority of all skin cancers in the US according to ACS. They usually never spread from one area of the body to the other. They appear like a dome-shaped bump with a pearly center, pink or red sore that reappears and bleed.** But if left untreated as they grow and invade the surrounding tissue, they cause damage as they enlarge. If caught early enough they can be excised with minimal, if any, recurrence or disfigurement.

Persons at risk of basal cell carcinoma:

- Anyone who has extensive sun exposure, especially to the face, ears, lips, arms, and shoulders
- Light- or fair-colored skin, light or red hair
- Persons with compromised immune systems, whether from disease or medication-induced, or a transplant patient may have ten times higher risk
- Persons with prior history of basal cell skin cancer

Squamous cell carcinoma (SCC): a skin cancer that begins in the squamous cells, which compose most of the skin's upper layers (the epidermis; these cells lie above the layer of basal cells, closest to the surface in the top layer of the piecrust). This skin cancer is more genetically complex, therefore can have more severe of an outcome if not detected early and properly treated. The lesions can occur in the same locations as basal cell carcinoma can. **The incidence of SCC of the skin has increased by more than 250 percent** since the 1970s. It is the most common skin cancer among African-Americans. SCC caused by sun exposure often look like crusted or scaly red patches, open sores, elevated growths with a central depression, or warts. They may crust or bleed.

Persons at risk for squamous cell carcinoma:

- Persons with extensive sun exposure
- Fair-skinned, light or red hair, blue, green or hazel, light eye color
- Usually occurs more often in men
- Persons with skin conditions or diseases not mentioned here, like actinic keratosis, actinic cheilitis, leukoplakia, and Bowen's disease
- All nationalities, as it can occur with history of extended sun exposure, so type of employment may play a role if outdoor work is involved
- Anyone with prior history of basal cell carcinoma
- Weakened and compromised immune systems from diseases or by medication, or transplant patients (have a sixty-five times higher risk)
- Usually young women with history of use of indoor tanning beds and or UV-sensitive
- Persons with severe skin damage from burns, ulcers, chronic infections or other injuries

When basal cell carcinoma and squamous cell carcinoma are found early and treated properly, there is a 95 percent cure rate for both types. See a dermatologist with any concerns.

Malignant Melanoma

The third type of skin cancer to be discussed is malignant melanoma. **It is the most serious skin cancer of all. Once a cell decides to take off to who knows where is when it is likely to become fatal.**

Malignant melanoma: This cancer starts with the melanocytes cells, which give the skin its color (these are found in the top piecrust layer closest to the surface, just as the squamous cells are found). Melanoma is a more serious type of skin cancer because it can spread to other parts of the body, by the lymphatic system or blood. Its main risk factor is ultraviolet radiation, whether it be from tanning beds or exposure to sunlight. The **appearance can vary**, but are usually flat or slightly raised discolored patch with irregular borders. They can be various colors—black, blue, brown, tan, or white. Usually found on the trunk of men, on the legs in women, or on the back of both men and women.

Malignant melanoma skin cancer is the most deadly form of skin cancer. It is the leading cause of all skin cancer-related deaths, and has a significantly lower five-year survival rates for its victims if it spreads to other areas of the body. Your physician can give you these survival rates, as sources will vary with percentage risk. Melanomas are not as common as basal cell and squamous cell skin cancers, but can be far more serious. Melanoma can almost always be cured in its early stages. This is why skin checks are so important.

Persons at risk for malignant melanoma skin cancer:

- Everyone with extensive exposure to UV radiation, whether by exposure to sunlight or other sources
- Persons who have used tanning beds that have UV radiation associated with them
- Fair-skinned persons, in accordance with Fitzpatrick skin photo-type scale, skin types 1 and 2
- Persons who freckle or sunburn easily, redheads or blond hair
- Persons with sun sensitivity or who have had painful blistering sunburns may also be at risk later in life
- The weekend tanners have a higher risk for melanoma than persons who are in the sun more regularly, like farmers or outdoor workers

- Persons with increased numbers of common and atypical moles on the body
- Persons with a family history of melanoma are more likely to develop skin cancer
- Older men have the highest incidence and mortality rates from malignant melanoma

The ABCDE's of Melanoma

A good way to help you remember the first signs are the **ABCDE's of Melanoma—Asymmetry, Borders, Color, Diameter, and Evolution.**

A = Asymmetry Melanoma are usually asymmetric. This means that one side of the mole looks different from the other. Ordinary moles are usually round or oval and symmetric (the same all around).

B = Borders Melanomas have uneven borders (edges) that are ragged, notched, or blurred. Ordinary moles have even borders.

C = Color Melanomas have uneven coloring. They may have patchy areas of brown, blue, red, tan, white, gray, or pink. Ordinary moles are usually an even shade of brown or tan.

D = Diameter Melanoma usually measure more than ¼ inch across (diameter). One-quarter inch (6mm) is about the size of a pencil eraser. Some melanomas are smaller. Ordinary moles are usually smaller than ¼ inch across and they stay the same size and shape over time.

E = Evolution Melanoma usually change in size, shape, or color over a short period of time. Ordinary moles stay the same size, shape, and color for many years.

Staging for Malignant Melanoma Cancer

There are also many cancer 'stages' for melanoma, and this depends on many factors. Accuracy in a diagnosis and classification for staging for melanoma is only established after the evaluation of the skin lesions' characteristics, both clinically and microscopically, are completed. They clinically note the evolution of the lesion, its location, size, depth, appearance, color, borders, and then a microscopic evaluation to include the rate in which it multiplies and how far its cells have spread in depth and width. As I mentioned earlier, staging is a collaborative effort by many different professionals: your managing physician, pathologist, radiologist, and cancer registrar all provide valuable staging information to your physician(s). Your physician has routine access to your personal history and all your pertinent information (biopsies, imaging studies, procedures, surgical findings) regarding your initial diagnosis. Your physician takes the lead in providing you with a 'staging' diagnosis for melanoma. Guidelines also change for staging. Your physician will be able to inform you.

Medical Pearl

The ABCDE's are a helpful way to remember the first signs of melanoma and what to watch out for in a freckle. Consult your physician if you are concerned about ANY skin change such as a new mole or change in the size or color of a preexisting mole.

CHAPTER THREE

IT IS ALL IN THE RAYS

WHAT ABOUT THE RAYS

I had so much information given me that once I read it and understood the significance of sunscreen that I felt I could share some basic information with you. The leading and world-renowned dermatologists are trying very hard to get the pharmaceutical companies to change the labels on the sunscreens you and I purchase. It will be a very slow process here in California. The thought is to make sure we the consumer understand what we are buying and what type of protection we are really getting. **The most important thing to remember when it comes to sunscreen is to APPLY the sunscreen in the first place.**

There is confusion amongst the public as to how much SPF do we really need to prevent skin cancer. Let me just say there is no SPF sunscreen in the world that will totally prevent the occurrence of skin cancer. According to the 2011 Melanoma Research Foundation and 2012 Skin Cancer Foundation, daily application of sunscreen may reduce the risk by slightly over half and possibly up to seventy percent. This doesn't sound like a lot, but it is a big deal. A minimum application of SPF 15 is suggested for daily use, but SPF of 30 is preferred, especially if in the sun for an extended period of time. We need to understand who is at risk and what potentially causes skin cancer to begin with. Then we can try and protect ourselves the best way possible and try to prevent it from occurring to the best of our ability. **Applying protection in the first place is key.**

Ultraviolet (UV) radiation rays are responsible for sunburns, aging of the skin, and skin cancer. There are two types of rays, **UVA** and **UVB.** Both do damage to the skin and promote aging. But one does more damage simply because of its intensity. The **UVA**-type rays, which are strong all day and all year long, are responsible for 95 percent of the UV radiation coming from the sun. The other, or **UVB**-type rays, penetrate the skin less deeply, but are 400 times more intense in the summer and in midday hours between 10:00 AM and 4:00 PM. The UVB rays compromise the other 5 percent of UV radiation. **The UVB rays play the biggest role in causing sunburns and all skin cancers.** But lately studies are indicating UVA rays play a role in accelerated aging of the skin and skin cancer. **So this being said, either avoid sun exposure during this 10:00 AM to 4:00 PM range, wear protective skin clothing with proper coverage, or apply sunscreen regularly and repeatedly during these intense peak hours. It is all you can do, those two options.**

The reality is a 20 percent chance you will get skin cancer in the course of your lifetime. This means: **One in five Americans will get skin cancer in their lifetime. This is with the nonmelanoma skin cancer types. Basal cell and squamous cell predominate, but malignant melanoma skin cancer is the most deadly form of skin cancer.**

Sunscreen Talk

What about sunscreen? In general, the following are the *biggest issues* when it comes to sunscreen:

1. We – **do not USE it** (SPF 15 or higher if in extensive sun exposure) in order to *aid* in prevention.
2. We – **do not use sunscreen properly**; this is one of the biggest issue because of 3, 4, and 5.
3. We – **do not apply enough to begin with.**

4. We – **do not reapply regularly while in the sun.**
5. We – **do not wait long enough before we enter the water to allow it to have maximum protection.**

One of the biggest problems is we do not apply enough in the first place and we don't let it sit on the skin long enough to penetrate the layers so it can be as effective as possible for us as the labeling suggests. Follow the directions on the bottle. We think we know, but reread the directions next time you apply sunscreen. Using it matters in aiding with prevention, but even this does not protect us 100 percent against skin cancers. **The key is finding a brand you like (SPF 15 or above) and using it regularly. A rule of thumb is to use two to three tablespoons for your body and one table-spoon for your face and reapply to both areas every two to four hours.** You must use this amount in order to achieve the SPF level in the product. If you apply less, then maybe your 30 SPF is really a lower SPF. Think about it. I have been informed there is no such thing as waterproof sunscreen. Applying it correctly in the first place does matter. **Always use a 30 SPF if in extensive sun hours.**

Labeling changes may be in the future to include broad-spectrum filters. Full UVA filtration has been harder to achieve in the US. A product with 'Anthelios' XL SPF 45 is what was recommended to me and I purchased it online from a pharmacy in Canada. The web site is http://www.pharmacymic.com. There are two other products you can search the web for sunscreens that contain a chemical called 'avobenzone' which is photo-stabilized with 'octocrylene' and provide the best in UVA protection. I was also informed to try and purchase Tinosorb, but it was not available on this site. They had several out-of-stock products. Also soon they are hoping to change labeling indicating 'water resistant' or 'very water resistant.' That will take a while and will depend upon how well they retain their SPF factor after water immersion. These products are more expensive than retailer prices.

General Key Points

- Apply a minimum sunscreen with SPF 15 or higher like 30, as directed on bottle daily before you go outside. **According to the SCF, the daily proper use of sunscreen reduced the risk of melanoma by slightly over 50 percent to 73 percent.**
- It is recommended a VIT D3 supplementation of 1,000 – 2,000 mg daily intake and it is much safer than sun exposure UV radiation rays. Both will raise seral VIT D3 levels. (Do not mistake VIT D3 with VIT D2: check your label.)
- Incidental sunlight is adequate for sufficient vitamin D levels in most fair-complexioned persons. Both will raise vitamin D levels.
- Avoid midday sun exposure: the 10:00 AM to 4:00 PM intense UVB rays peak time
- Avoid tanning practices, including tanning beds
- Wear hats, protective clothing, and sunglasses.

All of these are well-established practices in terms of reducing the photo-aging process and preventing skin cancer.

Medical Pearl for Women

So on a side note, being an OB-GYN nurse practitioner and as I would remind my patients: According to the NCI, **breast cancer is the most commonly diagnosed cancer in women worldwide, and the second leading cause of death in women, next only to lung cancer.** So why do you think performing your own monthly breast exams are so important? Because people who are diligent about their healthcare usually will see their physician once a year for ONE breast exam and that other female business. What about the other eleven months out of the year? Women, or their husband/partners, are more likely to pick up the change in a breast if they are doing their monthly self-breast exams, more so than their physician. So do your monthly self-breast exam as you have been taught. Touch them, get to know what they feel like, and don't forget to look at them also. **Discuss with**

your physician the signs of breast cancer so you can become more aware. One in eight (about 12 percent) women in the US will encounter breast cancer during her lifetime. Most breast cancers are diagnosed after the age of fifty. When I started practicing, the risk was one in twelve. So my advice to you: do your monthly self-breast exams (if you don't know how, ask your physician to teach you), keep up with your annual screenings, stay in a healthy weight zone, minimize your alcohol consumption, and never ever ignore a 'change.' It may save your life. "When in doubt, check it out," that is my motto. **See your physician right away if you have any concerns regarding your breasts.**

CHAPTER FOUR

ANOTHER MELANOMA LESION

Considering Options/SLN Biopsy

Once the biopsy results returned malignant melanoma for the second time, I knew my team of doctors was about to get larger. She referred me to one of her colleagues at Stanford who was responsible for discussing my options in more detail. I met with the director of the Dermatology and Melanoma Clinic who is also a professor of dermatology at Stanford Medical School. Stanford being a teaching hospital, there is always an additional intern or resident in the room as well, or an extra set of eyes, which I am fine with. The options were reviewed:

My first option: Complete surgical reexcision/resection of the lesion on my back and see what the pathology shows. This would be an in office procedure, with local anesthesia for numbing the area of concern. There are multiple injections to the site to get the area numb shallow and deep. Excision is done, the specimen is sent to the lab for microscopic evaluation and pathology. The procedure can take up to two hours or longer, depending on location and size. You can request a mild sedative prior to the procedure, which helped me the first go-around in 2013.

Second option: Complete surgical reexcision/resection of the lesion on my back, AND to include a sentinel lymph node (SLN) biopsy. This would be an outpatient surgery and under general anesthesia. The procedure would take about three to four hours. The big word is **lymphoscintigraphy, which just means sentinel lymph node mapping, or the first stop that drains a cancer.** As defined below.

The sentinel lymph node (SLN) is defined as the hypothetical 'first' lymph node or group of nodes (the amount of nodes varies from surgery to surgery and person to person) that the cancer cells are most likely to spread from a primary tumor or the lesion.

In this case, it was my melanoma skin lesion on my back. Malignant melanoma skin cancer has cancer cells within it and if the cells travel outside the lesion, most likely the first stop for them is the primary drainage site in the lymph system, which is a lymph node. Either option would 'be reasonable' and fine with her. SLN biopsy would give all of us more information whether the melanoma lesion had spread into my lymph nodes. **That is what the fear with malignant melanoma skin cancer is... the spreading of cancerous cells to other organs in the body via the lymphatic or circulatory system. This is where the real fight is and this is where the battle can be lost. Five-year survival rates drop significantly when it becomes invasive (meaning it has already spread to another organ). Your physician can inform you of your prognosis.**

I was quoted chances of it being in the lymph nodes to be less than 4 percent to 10 percent. More like 4 percent to 6 percent. It was my option, and I could decide. Either option would 'be reasonable.' That seemed to be the short phrase I would hear a lot in the next few months. But because it was the second lesion, the size of the lesion, I should consider it. I also mentioned the pain in my scapula area just prior to the lesion discovery, and I was convinced of its obvious association. That pain has to be linked to this melanoma lesion somehow. What should I do?

I had been so diligent about keeping my every-three-month dermatology appointments for three years. I've stayed proactive, tried to be preventative even. If we would proceed with the reexcision to include the SLN biopsy, this would keep us proactive and staying aggressive. This gave us as well as my team of physicians more knowledge. And more knowledge for better understanding of where you are with a diagnosis is always a good thing, right? After all, I had 94–96 percent chance all would be clear. I am going to prove the odds are correct. One would bet on those odds. Now, I am not going to take this decision lightly and nor should I. You ponder over the pros and cons incessantly. We had a small family discussion regarding the more involved surgery with our grown daughters. Both married and wonderful mothers. The discussion had to include the possible risks associated with this surgery, as this had been explained to me in detail. The risk was a 20 percent chance of swelling, infection, and possible loss of mobility or use of the arm, as nerves may be cut. If any of these risks occur, life would change somewhat for me, and a "new normal" in life would need to be understood. Especially with the possible loss of use of my arm. This would end up affecting all of us.

My new cutaneous oncology surgeon had said this could be a very manageable postoperative course. Her patients usually did very well, and this was her area of expertise. She had said she would locate and protect the two main nerves that allow complete movement in our arms and shoulders. It was her job to identify the nerves and preserve this function. We decided to stay proactive and aggressive. Keep ahead of this melanoma 'ghost.' After about two weeks of discussion back and forth, surgery was scheduled for late February. It would be about a three-and-a-half hour procedure under general anesthesia.

I should do this. I could do this. I am scared to do this. But I really felt I needed to do this. It would certainly provide more of a peace of mind to me and my family. I know their personalities and some would worry more than others. It was going to be a peace of mind for all of us. Thus, it will provide us all with additional knowledge to the extent/stage of this diagnosis. Some risk just has to be taken.

SLN Biopsy Procedure

The reexcision or resection of the lesion on the back is not difficult, except to make sure they clear the margins or borders surrounding the cancer. In making a wide-enough excision, I was expecting another four-to-five-inch scar on my upper back as a result. This length of a scar also makes it easier for the skin to be laced back together seamlessly. It is the SLN biopsy that is very technical. It is very involved specifying where the lesion is draining to. Isn't it amazing that every square inch of our body has specific "draining zones," especially during an injury or infection?

There are syringes filled with radioactive substance, a blue dye, and these are injected near the tumor site. Injections may be given at all four corners of the lesion. There is a waiting period for the cellular activity to do its thing, and then a radiology scan to confirm it has traveled to the area for detection. The mapping of where the lesion would drain could have been to my groin, my neck, or my axillary (armpit) area. This mapping can be different for every person even if the lesion is in the same area. Then you are immediately taken into surgery where a Geiger counter-like piece of equipment is used to pick up the radioactivity. The blue dye makes it visible to the surgeon, and this is where the focus for the surgical biopsy is done. It is at this point where the surgeon will decide how many lymph nodes 'light up' that she feels need removal for pathological evaluation. When this procedure is done, everyone's mapping for a specific area of their body to drain may be different but will be identified.

Surgery Day for SLN Biopsy

So as my second malignant melanoma lesion is confirmed in February 2017, the decision is made to do the complete reexcision of the lesion, which will include the sentinel lymph-node biopsy surgery. Now I just want to get on with it. The surgeon stated she usually will take about three or so lymph nodes out for diagnostic purposes, and she expected that area of the lesion would most likely drain to my axilla (armpit).

My surgery had to be rescheduled and pushed back one week as I was getting over pneumonia. It had originally been scheduled for Valentine's Day. The wait was so difficult once a decision had been made. I let my family and friends know of the upcoming surgery and requested prayers for a successful procedure and outcome. I felt the genuine concern from all. Prayers were being sent up all across the country, as my husband had all his support system with his coworkers in prayer as well. There is comfort knowing others are praying for you, and small prayer groups were keeping me in their thoughts also. One can never underestimate the power of prayer.

It is surgery day today, February 21, 2017. As with any inpatient surgery, I needed to go through the preadmitting routine and provide insurance information. I head to my preop room and get ready with a beautiful gown to wear. A warm pair of socks, blanket, and a beautiful shower cap added to the wardrobe and I am ready for the runway, on a gurney. All the routine questions have been asked and the consent is signed reminding me of all the horrible things that may go wrong. So—I sign it. The intravenous line is started, and it takes one or two tries to get it going—ouch—but I am not changing my mind on this. They get the fluids going and now I am officially ready for the operating room.

As the process for the SLN biopsy was explained in lighter detail by my surgeon, I needed to understand how this was going to go. Some people do not like knowing the details or particulars, but I do. There is nothing wrong with either preference: everyone is different. I am sure it is my curious medical mind. In my case the lesion being on my back, the injection with dye goes into the back around the lesion, and then the scan is done while we wait for the material to travel to its primary lymph node site. I thought *Perhaps this would all be done while I was under anesthesia. My goodness, we have to be brave. The nuclear medicine team knows the procedure and are ready to get started. I am at the mercy of the doctors, and I am praying this radiologist has done hundreds of these before.* Some hands are more experienced than others, and I just decided it is a bit too late to ask. What difference was it going to make now? Behind the procedure room window, I could see several eager young faces that I could only assume are doctors-in-training. So, just to be clear and repeat this procedure back to the radiologist, "You need to inject me with those syringes in my back four times while I lay still and awake?" He said, "Yes, at each of the four corners of the lesion site, but there is only a small amount of material that needs to be injected." My husband was sitting in the far corner of the room; I glanced at him and asked if he felt he could watch this or would he need to step out. He said he would be fine. I thought for a moment on what I was about to go through, and then just turned over on my stomach. I realize I have endured worse with the in-office excision the first time! You can't be brave unless there is an element of fear in you. I had an element of fear. Okay, let's get this done. I recited over and over in my head while he was injecting me, "*Be still, and know that I am God, be still and know that I am God.*" Where will my primary site be? As that will be the target for the sentinel lymph node dissection. I will not know until surgery is over and I feel for a bandage. Why is the lymph node so important?

What is the Lymphatic System?

The lymphatic system: refers to the organs and tissues, including lymph nodes and bone marrow, that make, store, and carry lymph cells; these cells fight infections and other diseases.

The lymphatic system provides approximately 10 percent of our circulatory system, with our blood vessels providing the other 90 percent. The number of lymph nodes varies depending on which source you look at. Some sites state we have over 800 total, others say we have approximately 500–700 lymph nodes in our body. **The number of lymph nodes in our body varies from individual to individual**. About half of the nodes are in the middle of our body (stomach or abdominal cavity). The largest grouping of lymph nodes are found in the neck, our armpits, and groin areas. The amount of nodes in the axillary region varies with approximately 20 to 40, in two clumps, and sit at varying depths within the site. These are little depot areas, basins, or stations if you will.

The lymphatic system is intertwined with the circulatory system. The blood circulation is a CIRCULAR system that moves nutrients to cells in the body and removes wastes from the tissue cells. The wastes are then carried to the liver, kidneys, and lungs so they can be excreted. However, some of the cell waste are larger molecules that cannot be removed by the blood. This is where the lymph system comes in. It is responsible for removing the rest of these wastes. It is a ONE-WAY system that picks up these large waste molecules and a lot of water molecules from the tissues of the body, and carries them to the larger blood vessels so the waste can be removed.

Basically, what the two-way system cannot handle the one-way system handles the job in carrying the bigger waste molecules from the cells in the tissues to the larger vessels for excretion. The kidneys, liver, and lungs are the body's organs that help with this complete process.

The lymph fluid is a clear liquid with a slightly yellow tinge, and is sticky. Very much like the fluid that comes out when you pop a blister. It is made up of the waste protein molecules, water molecules that attract the proteins and bits of dead and broken down cells, foreign cells such as bacteria, viruses, fungus cells, and anything else that does not belong in the body, such as perfumes and chemicals. So while it plays a role in carrying all the impurities out of the body and travels from organ to organ, you can see how it may carry the cancer cells (which would be considered foreign cells) to otherwise healthy organs, hence the spread has just occurred. This is when the battle becomes more difficult to win.

So the lymph system has an important role aiding in boosting our immune system. Meaning—helping us stay healthy. Therefore, when lymph nodes have been removed, the immune system is compromised. The extent of compromise depends on the amount of lymph nodes that have been damaged or have been excised. The more nodes removed, most likely the more insult to our immune system. This system helps fight infections, heal injuries, and all plays an integral part of the body's attacking system.

As my surgeon explained, it something similar and to the effect: "They are like little pearls encased in butter." The 'butter' is really adipose tissue or fatty tissue. You need to scoop the butter out, melt it down to see the quality of the pearls. Then the pearls are dissected and under microscopic examination, the cells are identified. The verdict: one way or the other, cancerous or not, can then be made. Depending on how many need removal, they are carefully extracted from the site, with some major skill and patience required here. Highly impressive surgical achievement.

The radiologist portion of the procedure would take almost 30 to 45 minutes, including the scan to track the primary draining site, and you cannot let the time get away from you. After a routine prayer moment with my husband, I am wheeled into the operating room. I am still, and I know He will be here with me.

SLN Biopsy Surgery Goes Well

Surgery went well and was about a three-and-half-hour procedure. It went without complications. As I slowly awoke, I noticed I had a bandage under my left armpit area. I also immediately lifted my arm and was able to do so. I was thankful for this. The surgeon had taken three axillary lymph nodes for diagnostic purposes, to see if the melanoma had spread. The reexcision on my back went well. It is about a four-and-a-half-inch scar, but scars do not bother me—yet. I had yet to experience that deep inner chest pain that I had complained about prior to the biopsy being taken again. The incision under my arm was pretty lengthy as well, about four to five inches. We made the trip home and during the following week, I experienced some intense pain in both incision sites for a couple of weeks. Tylenol seemed to take care of my discomfort, and I preferred not take any narcotics after this surgery. My throat is what hurt the most—I could hardly talk. That took almost a week to feel better. I would guess they must have some difficulty getting the endotracheal tube/breathing tube in: I checked and it took three times. But after one week, my wounds were healing very nicely.

We, my family, had talked all week about staying positive and focusing on the greater than ninety-four percent chance it would NOT be in my lymph nodes. After all, initial pathology showed it was a Stage I-A lesion, again. We welcomed the continued prayers, and I really tried to stay positive and strong. Strong for my family and my husband. I was in routine prayer as well, but had not started journaling as yet, and the inspiration for this book had not been even been a thought. But—and sometimes there is a "but"!— no matter how hard I tried, something deep down inside was gnawing at me. I don't know exactly what or why. Maybe just natural humanistic worry with something of this magnitude, and such devastating and frightening statistics if this ends up in my lymph nodes. BUT my gut was telling me something else. I could not shake the feeling, and kept it to myself.

One-week follow-up appointment

We traveled to my appointment on March 1, 2017 and that feeling in my gut just would not go away. Was it just normal worry and a nervous stomach? Possibly. My surgeon's nurse, who said she would call me with the negative results, fell silent all week. We entered the exam room. Vital signs were taken, my blood pressure was up—really. The nurse entered the room and I said, "Hello, we are here for some good news!" She made a mention my doctor was on the phone with another physician and would be in shortly. So we all waited together and made small talk.

The exam room door opened slowly and my surgeon, who appeared no older than my own daughter, poked her head in and entered the room gingerly. I said, "Okay, we have some good news today?" I was trying to show my husband I was staying positive, as I had all week.

She spoke softly and said, "Well, I have some good news and some bad news."

At that very moment, I knew what my gut was telling me was right. At that point, I couldn't even glance at my precious husband who is always by my side. We have been together since the age of fifteen and we married right before my twentieth birthday. Who does that anymore? Forty-three years together and I am so thankful and blessed. He absolutely just hates anything associated with hospitals, period, but he sat there quietly and listened.

My surgeon continued, "First, the good news: we got the entire melanoma lesion excised with wide margins from your back. But the bad news is there is a micrometastasis in one of three of the sentinel lymph nodes." So ... one in three of the lymph nodes had a micro amount of melanoma cancer cells within it. Remember it all starts with one single cell. Microscopic amount. Hmmm. Still a positive finding: in the lymph nodes, but the outcome is better? This was an early catch for sure. I still don't feel very good, though; the pit in my stomach just validated what my biggest fear would be. I have cancer. I felt one tear slowly stream down my cheek as I tried to understand how a Stage I lesion could lead to this. I had over 94 percent chance this would not happen. What? I hate, yes, hate, being on this end of the playing field, as everyone does.

The news is a game changer. The treatment plan will now require more decisions, and they will be much tougher decisions. More physicians need to be involved, and more appointments need to be made. Now I have to meet back with the melanoma lead physician to explain this new development in more detail and review all the option plans. An oncologist will be assigned to me. Wait, what has just happened? The word "high-risk" kept running through my head. Is this real?

Again, I do recognize I have not received the 'worst of the worst' news, and I am thankful for this. But this is fresh news and I am trying to process it all. This is truly a scare to say the least. To think that in a short period of time it had traveled into the lymphatic system. Was the deep pain in my chest related to this finding? The 'one' cell going rogue, I don't know. But what I do know is I went from Stage I-A to Stage III-A overnight. What happened here? This lesion was smaller than the first melanoma lesion. I am in shock. What would have happened had I not done the sentinel lymph node dissection in the first place? How am I going to tell my daughters—I have cancer?

So this must be what 'fear' feels like.

Spiritual Pearl ~ One

My faith being tested has brought about my spiritual revival. I didn't know how deep my faith really was, but I already knew that I have not been the Christ follower He would want me to be with my breadth of knowledge in this area. Since my medical journaling has not yet begun, I write as I think back on this timeframe for me in two areas. Number one—awaiting to get this surgery over with, and two—waiting for the results of my SLN biopsy. The biggest impact for deciding to move forward with the SLN biopsy came from my dermatologist who had said to me; "Sometimes you have to be willing to take the risks in order to gain in knowledge." Think about that for a minute. Weighing the risk associated with the SLN biopsy as mentioned earlier, with gaining in knowledge for a more conclusive diagnosis and therefore direct and individualized treatment plan. This knowledge could prove to be bad news or good news. But at least I would know where

I stand with my complete diagnosis. I would soon realize I could no longer manipulate or control any of my circumstances, so my faith must be placed in someone other than myself. My team of physicians would play a role in this for sure. I remind myself and choose God to be my Chief of Staff.

So I decided to gain in knowledge and learn more about what it means to have faith. My resources would help point me in the right direction, so as not to be overwhelming. It can be a daunting task thinking I have to be versed in the bible. But at the 'risk' of being embarrassed of how naïve I am with my biblical walk, with God's grace the baby steps I took led me to gain in knowledge which infused my soul. So I started my biblical education slowly, hoping it would guide me to discover more about what depth of faith means to me. I would look up the scripture associated with the daily devotional I was reading and took notes on it if it so moved me. I found I began focusing on five words: Faith, Trust, Peace, Hope, and Joy. So these became my 'strength' words. At the same time, these were baby steps for me. God is so patient and His grace is warming. Like everything about Him.

> "So we fix our eyes not on what is seen, but what is unseen. Since what is seen is temporary, and what is unseen is eternal."
>
> 2 COR 4:18

> "We live by Faith, not by sight"
>
> 2 COR 5:7

God already knows my circumstance and how it will unfold. He may choose not to remove this trial from me, even though He could. All the while, He has a perfect plan laid out for me. The qualities that I will need to help strengthen me for all eternity will be instilled in me spiritually during this time. And there will be many lessons I will learn, however this unfolds. I would gain in knowledge here, for a clearer path immediately. I need to walk by faith and not by sight. We are not called to go through these trials alone, in our walk of faith. At this time, I say, as some of us have said before, 'Thank God.'

CHAPTER FIVE

IT IS ALL IN THE DELIVERY

DELIVERING BAD NEWS

I have been an OB-GYN nurse practitioner with a second specialty in reproductive endocrinology-infertility for over twenty-seven years—basically specializing in women's health. Through the years, I have worked with some very knowledgeable physicians from whom I learned many valuable lessons. I have been exposed to a variety of diagnosis and health conditions, and have witnessed both joyous and devastating outcomes. I have had to deliver challenging news to some of my patients, as well as joyous news over the years. Whether it was good news or bad, it may have affected both the young and old. All the while when delivering the news, I wanted to sound empathetic, confident, and encouraging, so as to provide hope and guidance for treatment options. Ultimately when there are options, it's their decision. But I think my patients would say that I did not 'sugarcoat' my concerns. Some may even say, 'How could she say "that," as it's tough to hear.'

Sometimes there are no options. For instance, there is no option when a heart stops beating in an embryo or fetus while in utero, as I experienced. It can occur in any trimester for a variety of reasons. Sometimes there is no known reason as to 'why' this happens. The 'why' in this case is what every mother wants an answer to. It is tough to hear the words, "We don't know" as an answer, and "We may never know." On occasion, we can tell what the probable cause may have been, or it is very evident as to be the cause. Doing cultures or an ultrasound may aid in revealing the truth or it may be determined only after delivery is made. But the truth is we may never have an answer.

So how a stage I melanoma lesion got into my lymph nodes we do not know. The lymph system carries "foreign cells" to the bigger vessels to be excreted from the body. So where exactly am I sitting in this process of the lymph system getting the job done? A melanoma cell just went rogue—are there more somewhere? The answer: 'We do not know.' But either way we cannot reverse the devastating circumstance of a heartbeat that has stopped and make life resume at that time, or reverse that cancer cell from going solo. No matter what trimester it is, there is no other option but delivery. The only options to discuss would be the delivery method: await for a spontaneous delivery (sometimes this isn't even an option), induced delivery, or surgical delivery. What a devastating decision to be made, when it is supposed to be one of the most exciting and joyous experiences in life. This is all part of life, that trek which does not promise to be a painless one. Those who have endured the loss of a baby or experienced a miscarriage will never forget exactly what they went through. It is a circumstance beyond our control. Most mothers can recount it all. They can feel the pain it left behind right in the center of their heart.

Just as there is no option when you inform a woman who wants to conceive a child, a biological child, and it's unlikely because she is in premature menopause (ovarian failure) at the age of thirty-two. She can be a mother, but not a biological mother, for she can no longer produce an ova (egg). A circumstance again beyond anyone's control.

Delivering bad news is not a comfortable position to be in, but it is part of a medical provider's job. Some news is much tougher to deliver than other news, and I know some of it is very difficult to hear. I can tear up easily when I recall some of the news I've had to deliver in the past. I have shared many tears with some of my patients, and even after they leave my office it can take me a while to absorb the news. Some of my patients were my age when I started in women's health, and they have stayed with me for over twenty-plus years. My last seven years of practice, as I mentioned earlier, has been in the health center at a local state college, as the GYN health specialist; their time is more limited and they move on. I have had to deliver news on various levels there as well. So circumstances beyond our control is when the emotional turmoil can peer in and we are suddenly very unprepared. But now the shoe is on the other foot for me. Again I do not feel comfortable in this position, nor in these shoes.

After I heard the news of the cancer making its way into my lymph nodes, the sudden onset of anxiety-driven physical symptoms became noticeable. The turmoil began: I became aware of my heart starting to race, my face was feeling hot and flushed, my palms were sweating and at times my hands felt very cold. Now I have a different sense of empathy for all of my patients in the past who had to hear any kind of news from me! The 'delivery' of challenging news is so important. It is all in the delivery. Actually, the 'delivery' in anything tough that requires discussion is a talent in itself. We must be honest, and bad news does happen, especially in medicine. The delivery does not make the fear or worry of what is to come subside. But the 'delivery' can show that the provider cares.

I felt my doctor was being straight with me and, at the same time, I felt she was giving me hope for an optimistic outcome. Her delivery carried empathy and concern. She was very knowledgeable and encouraging. But the fact did remain this was cancer. No matter how small it was, it was not insignificant. No one could be sure it was not anywhere else in my body. I asked questions to everyone involved, "How do we know that was all there was in the lymph nodes?" "Can we be sure it is not in any other lymph nodes?" This 'ghost' of an amount. This question would not be answered. It was a "we don't know" answer. But it was not to be ignored, and now this changes everything. It is out of my control. Time will be the deciding factor.

After she delivered the bad news to me and as I tried to process it all, I began my dialogue with my surgeon: "Thank you for your excellent surgical skills, and I know this is not what any of us was expecting." Yes, I really did say this. It just came out. I realized as we were talking I had one tear stream down my cheek and so did her nurse. We spoke of what comes next. I still couldn't bear to glance at my husband, feeling the need to truly understand what this all meant. I needed to explain it to my family and this is not my area of expertise. After the initial shock, I did not want to miss anything, so it was almost as if we were discussing a different patient for a moment, and I needed to learn about this.

They stepped out of the room so referrals could be made. The room fell silent, and in the few seconds that followed there was only the beating of two hearts that could be heard, two hearts that had become one long ago. I remember sitting there for a few seconds and then getting up to hug my husband once the team left the exam room. In disbelief, I said "Why couldn't the good news and bad news have been reversed?" I remember saying this a few more times in the week ahead. Why couldn't they have needed to resect more off my back, but the lymph nodes all have been negative? After all, that is what the odds were. We were betting on the odds and hoping for the odds to prove accurate. But why was this happening?

I believe with all my heart—this is why! On March 7, 2017, I would start my days in prayer and began reading scripture on a more regular basis. I had not done this before for much length of time. I had not asked the question "Why couldn't the news be reversed?" again. You cannot know the strength of your faith until it is truly tested. Just how important is my walk of faith to me? That is the real question, and this was the real moment. He is watching me. He is waiting for me. He is longing for a visit, my visit. And He already knows me by name.

And so it began. I have been tested. My entire family has been tested. Just how strong is our faith now? Even though I was reading more spiritual literature, I had not started actually writing my emotional experience or thoughts down in my little pink journal for almost two months later, after the next step of treatment. The reality remains I am worried, and I am fearful. I do not know what will happen next. I do not know how this is all going to end. My sister had said to me once, "You never know when you are one doctor's appointment away from news that will change your life." The next-step decisions to be made will not only impact me, but also all those I love dearly. And yes, it changed my life.

The results of this pathology made this appointment a lengthy one. I had several missed text messages from family and friends wanting to know the update and waiting for me as I turned my phone back on. We decided to drive to my youngest daughter's home first to discuss the report, as it was on the way home anyway. We would call my eldest daughter from her house. We discussed on the drive over that I would play with our two granddaughters and keep them entertained while my husband, who seemed to grasp more than I thought, would deliver the news. We were certain there would be tears, and there were. My daughters are thirty-three and thirty-four years old. They are amazing women, daughters, wives, and mothers. They are my best friends. We are a tight family unit I would say. We raised them as Christians and they do believe there is a God. Even through the college years they maintained their faith. They may not have gone to church every Sunday while they were in college, nor as young mothers, but they never waived in their belief. They have chosen spouses who are believers also.

If I was not a believer, I do not know if I would have reached out in the direction of 'developing a faith' for encouragement and strength. For the majority of people, support from loved ones in situations like this is certainly there. I am not suggesting that if you are not a believer you could not possibly get through the challenges that lay ahead of you. Nor am I saying you would not be able to cope with receipt of news that is life-changing. For no matter what and for the believer or the nonbeliever, the battle in tackling this cancer challenge will follow for both of us, and it is waiting and looming overhead. For either of us, it is when the challenge has resolved, where our hope lies with regaining our good health in becoming cancer-free that remains the quest. I guess it is how the journey will unfold that becomes the trek for each of us. It will be our personal experience and a new chapter in our book of life.

It would be about five weeks later, or after the news of positive SLN biopsy but prior to my second surgery, that I picked up the little 'pink journal' and began jotting down my spiritual thoughts. Now I had kept my scriptural notes separate, on my legal pad, but I would date every entry so I could correlate the scriptural readings to my spiritual writings. This has helped with turning the totality of this experience into a very visual picture for me, and eventually the Holy Spirit within me pressed me to consider writing a book.

CHAPTER SIX

REFLECTING AND INVESTING IN THE WORD

MY FIRST 'PINK' JOURNAL ENTRY

This was my first journal entry and it started to flow on a beautiful spring morning. April 2, 2017. The concept of actually writing this book would come many months later. So I journaled as I felt moved, until one day something just happened. I cannot even explain it. I was hearing a call from within my soul and it took time for me to understand why, and in time I would figure out how I was going to accomplish it. But when you have the Holy Spirit encouraging you along, it kind of just falls into place. When the inspiration came, hopefully you will see and feel 'the why' I wanted to share this with you. So I write about my experience in my journal, it unfolded and slowly morphed into this. Portions of this book are heavily sprinkled with occasional excerpts from scripture readings or quotes I became attached to. In recovering from my recent surgery it begins, my baby steps….

April 2, 2017. As I sit here and write for the first time, on this peaceful Sunday morning, my husband attends our church service. A Sunday morning, how appropriate. I have been trying to spend more time with My God, My Father. Build on my breadth of scripture knowledge for my own reward. So, I open my daily devotional and I read about the Promise of My God to meet all my needs. Not just some, but ALL my needs according to His glorious riches. I needed to understand that during times of trouble, I needed to be thanking Him, for the peace I will find during this upcoming trial is supposed to far outweigh the trial truly awaiting me. This is a promise that He will be relentless in keeping.

So I guess this entry suggests the strength and peace I would gain during 'my challenge' will gradually be felt as I sit and quiet myself to get to know Him. Spend time with Him. In just a few short weeks of making this my morning routine, I am in awe of His majestic gifts, His teaching skills, and the comfort knowing I am not a stranger to Him. He wants to visit with me always. The hours pass swiftly when I am visiting. The word 'peace' has taken on a whole new meaning for me. It is so much more powerful and grand than the calm or serenity it suggests. It can be transforming. The struggle of this challenge will be real, but my heart can be calmed by this abundantly rich and glorious gift which His Peace promises to bring me.

The time in prayer for myself and my family had begun. The 'what ifs' crept into my mind. While trying to stay positive, I am also human. In the many days and nights ahead, I would notice the ebbs and flow of my emotional state from being scared of knowing what lies ahead, to being at peace in a single moment. It was a very different place for me to be, so uncertain. It was uncomfortable and comfortable.

IS THIS FEAR

There are so many moments during the day in the weeks ahead, awaiting my future appointments, when my heart would pound and my throat felt so tight. At times I felt I could hardly swallow. The tension in my shoulder and neck is a typical reaction to stress for me. I could feel the muscles in my upper back knotting up and getting tighter and tighter. My stomach would have this gnawing feeling and sometimes I just felt nauseated. I remember my hands would tremble on occasion. I could feel the welling of tears off and on throughout the day. Anxious times for sure. What can I do not to just fall apart knowing what decisions I have looming before me? I do not allow myself to dwell in the negative for very long. I never have, but this worry is occupying my thoughts a little more than usual. That overwhelming feeling is suddenly sprinkled in my daily life and is very real to me. My husband could sense my worry and sent me a scripture verse he thought would help me. So I memorized it, then recited it over and over when I could catch these moments creeping into my day. It was my 'go to.' God was always my "Go To." It may have taken me some time to remember that, but I eventually would get there.

> *"The Lord is near. Do not be anxious about anything, but in everything, by prayer and petition, with thanksgiving, present your requests to God. And the peace of God, which transcends all understanding, will guard your hearts and mind in Christ Jesus,"*
>
> Phil. 4:5–7

Reciting this in prayer would help me calm my thoughts as well as my heart in the many weeks ahead. I would cling to this throughout the days and nights. The nights are tough to sleep through uninterrupted, as I would get anxious and feel my heart race. Sometimes I would be awake for an hour or two at a time and would have difficulty getting back to sleep. So I would recite my Philippians 4: 5–7 over and over until I could fall asleep.

Spiritual Pearl ~ Two

I found it interesting that the word 'guard' your hearts and minds was used in that scripture. Why not 'guide' your hearts and minds? At the time I felt I needed guidance, preferred it. Someone just take my hand and lead me and make it all better. But 'to guard' means 'watch over in order to *protect* or *control.*' 'To guide' means 'to *lead, conduct, direct, or steer,* have influence on the course of action.' I love that the word 'guard' was used. It expresses concern and references to protection of your heart and mind. To control the racing of thoughts and the pounding of our hearts. It is during distress and under duress that we have physical symptoms and feel this way. He knows our body's response mechanisms to fear and to worry. He already knows. He created us. I had so many family and friends who kept me in their thoughts and prayers as I kept them updated on my health issue. Christian or not, all are special and all are blessings to me and would guard my heart.

LIFE GOES ON

In the midst of this news of malignant melanoma cancer for me, life does not stop. I had been dealing with a breast issue that I could not neglect. In September of 2016, I had an inflammatory reaction of my right breast, probably from an insect bite, but I wasn't sure this was the cause. I recalled a windy day on the college campus, and I was coming in from lunch with a friend of mine when some sort of beetle flew in my blouse and must have bitten me before I could swipe it out. It was a couple of days later, maybe longer, when I awoke one morning with my breast swollen and was lobulated and irregular in shape. I had ongoing redness, tenderness, induration (hardening of otherwise soft tissue), swelling of the breast (almost twice the size of my normal breast) and an abscess formation that was about the size of a thumb. I experienced excruciating pain, and wearing a bra was unbearable. I was referred to a general surgeon locally. I had a 3D mammogram, diagnostic breast ultrasound, weeks of antibiotics, in-office biopsies, and general surgery mid-November to drain the abscess which included more biopsies.

It took twenty-one agonizing days from the first visit to the testing, to the final diagnosis of "sterile abscess" and "negative for breast cancer." The week after this breast surgery in November was tough on my husband and me, as we would not have news for one week. Being a GYN nurse practitioner, my mind was reeling with the possible diagnosis of inflammatory breast cancer. I never mentioned this to my husband until the few days before my follow-up appointment. He knows me well, and noticed I looked really worried. I was much quieter than usual. We shed tears in the back-yard, and with thoughts of this ending with bad news. We were in prayer, but again it did not grip me in the spiritual engagement I have found myself in now. I would have to say fear is a powerful monster. Most of the time it is a monster of a lot of "nothing." Fear can be paralyzing. A big, paralyzing clump of dark–nothing–monster.

This is a breast cancer many women may not have heard of. This breast cancer does not have the typical "lump" to be found. With inflammatory breast cancer, the average age for onset is fifty-seven—I was fifty-seven. The sequence of symptoms that appear were exactly like the sequence that mine came in. It is an inflammatory reaction much like an infectious response. The survival rate is forty percent, a devastating survival rate. The breast cancer with lumpectomies, if caught early enough, may have 90 to 95 percent survival rate.

In mid-November 2016, when surgery was finally scheduled (and I know my surgeon had this in the back of her mind also), I actually said, "We are planning on ruling out IBC (inflammatory breast cancer)?" "That's the goal," she replied. Surgery went well, the usual. After the surgery, we did not hear a word from her office all week regarding results. Then the morning of my one week follow-up appointment, they called to cancel it—for whatever reason. These things happen: there are emergencies or illnesses that occur. I get it, but I told the nurse I needed a phone call today from someone, as I had been waiting all week for news of the biopsies. They called back thirty minutes later and said she wanted to see me in thirty minutes.

The drive to her office was quiet. Waiting is so hard, isn't it? Our minds spin, our hearts race and pound so hard that surely anyone standing next to us could hear it. And God knows we will react this way, if we can only include Him in our concerns and let Him carry the burden. The first thing she said was, "Well, everything is negative." She mentioned that surgery may be needed again if the abscess does not shrink in size, but time is what is needed for my 'girl' to heal up and return to normal. My immune system should aid my body and absorb the remainder of the abscess, but it will take time. I would continue with antibiotics and see her every three months for the progress on this moderately large breast abscess. When I followed up with her in January, I informed her of my recent news of malignant melanoma and that more options were being discussed. I mentioned most likely another surgery was in my near future. All this was going on at once. Obviously the fact this was not breast cancer was a very welcomed gift. I did thank God.

When this inflammation began and the fear of it being breast cancer crept in, we as a family did pray. In fact we prayed several times a day. My daughters, other family members and friends, their church groups, were sending up prayers. My family could definitely sense my worry. I was not myself. I was quieter and had a look of concern on my face, I guess all the time. I felt alone and afraid that this was going to be my battle. Let me be clear: I did not dwell in this all day long as I had distractions with work and household duties, but almost daily the fear of this would creep in and out. My sleeping habits were interrupted. There was 'worry' bouncing around in my head, and she brought her friend 'fear' with her.

My daughter Kendyl heard the song by Jason Gray, "The Sparrow." The song is based on the verse in the NKJV Bible in the book of Matthew 10:28–30. She had managed to go on Etsy, and have some of the lyrics written and then placed a sparrow, as if in flight, right in the center of the page and had it framed. She gave this to me as a gift, and it became a constant reminder that my God knows me. I am not alone.

"Are not two sparrows sold for a copper coin? And not one of them falls to the ground apart from your Father's will. But the very hairs on your head are all numbered,"

MATTHEW 10: 28–30

It took almost three months of antibiotics off and on, 3D mammogram, multiple breast ultrasounds, three breast biopsies, and general surgery. One year later as I sit here writing this here and now, my breast is finally healthier. Still, even with this awful breast scare and all the praying I did—we all did—it did not bring me to INVEST in the 'maturing' of my faith by spending time with Him. I can't mature in my faith if I don't invest in time reading the Word. I am a Christian, a believer, but I am not in a relationship with Him. We were so relieved with this news. Maybe, as we have all heard before, we don't think of God when things are going good—right? We pray when we are scared and afraid that things may go south or have gone south. It would take another week for me to realize I needed Him more. But was it the prayers that made the outcome the difference here? I don't know. Maybe. Possibly. I'll ask Him when I see Him.

INVESTING IN THE WORD

I still could not believe I went from Stage I to Stage IIIA overnight. Has there been a mistake in the lab? This went through my mind several times in fact. So I did ask, and all had been double-checked according to my physician. I had been praying off and on since September, when my breast scare popped up. But I had not been investing or relying on my faith. I was trusting and relying on my husband to provide a spiritual strength for me. He is so well-read and versed in the bible. But while he provided me with love and support, I see now it was not fair that I relied on him to supply the strength I needed when it came to my faith. This avenue for managing my fears or guarding my heart and mind was not working. It – was - not - working! To start walking by faith and not by sight is a difficult concept for some to grasp, but it must start from within yourself and not someone else in order to feel its value. We look for explanations in everything. Sometimes there is no explanation as to the 'why' things happen. But I realized as I look back that there was so much I was missing out on with spending time investing in the God I do in fact love. It was the 'trust' that was missing. Trust would become the channel through which His peace flows through me. I need trust.

My head was spinning and my concern was not only for myself but for my family and my employer as well. I knew there was going to be more chal-lenges ahead. It might be a tougher fight than I can imagine. How would this affect my husband, each one of my adult children, my work, and everything else in my life? Where would each of them find their support as I knew they would search as well? How would they find their strength? When would I even get back to work? Would I go back to work? After all I am fifty-seven, having been in medicine for thirty-seven years and women's health for over thirty. Would I give it up now and should I let it go? Would I be given a different path? Would I feel called to do something else? So many questions. Worrying, waiting, and hoping for an answer. I needed clarity. Turns out it would be circumstances known only to God. I would have to wait and do the best I could with what was ahead of me.

This is when I began reading and taking notes on the book, *The Strength You Need*. I would begin reading in my morning quiet time and, before I knew it, two to three hours had passed. I was a sponge—"engrossed" would be an understatement. Each chapter guided my path to understanding 'the why.' We will all experience trials in this life, but how we choose to navigate through them is a different story. When I turned my efforts into discovering more about my Lord, I did not know His burden would include alleviating my ailments promoted by worry and fear. I chose to focus more on Him and less on myself when I did not know what else to do. Slowly and timely, the encouragement and relief I found in my time with Him would begin my rescue from myself. He uses all kinds of trials in our lives to seek our attention. I can see this now. He wants me but He doesn't need me.

Just one week ago I had a three-hour appointment with physicians that I thought should not be in my life at this time. Now I know some of you may be saying, *Talk to me when your struggle is as hard as mine*. We can always think of someone, or even know someone, who has been dealt a worse hand. And there is always someone worse off than we are. No matter how difficult life is, someone else's pain may be greater and more devastating than our own. But identifying with this is probable.

Holy Spirit Moment ~ One

My days began to feel like they were running into each other, as I had one appointment after another. The wait after the surgery to hear results seemed like a very long time, when in reality it had been only seven days. There were definitely restless days and sleepless nights even as I tried so hard to stay positive. But as the news was revealed to me and the results were positive, I knew I needed to have a local oncologist as part of my medical team. So I inquired around, decided on one, and made an appointment. About one week later, which was about the same time I dove into some readings, I had an appointment. I chose one who would use the same electronic medical record system and would have access to my Stanford medical information, test results, office visits notations, etc. Anything to try and make it easier on myself.

So while on my drive to meet with my local oncologist for our first visit, I was feeling a little overwhelmed with so much on my plate. Some things remained unresolved in my breast and therefore open-ended, and I needed to stay on top of that issue. For the reality may be that I needed the abscess redrained, which meant surgery again. I was already thinking of how I could kill two birds with one stone and possibly have this done, if needed, at the same time with my next scheduled 'big' surgery. I also had just recovered from mycoplasma pneumonia and was finally treated with an antibiotic that could knock it out. That went on for eight to ten weeks or so, and extreme fatigue was associated with it. I was already so exhausted going into this next phase of treatment for melanoma. My first surgery to reexcise the melanoma lesion with the SLN biopsy actually had to be rescheduled for two weeks later, due to my lingering cough and fever spikes.

So many appointments had to be scheduled to discuss the next step or plan of action in more detail for my skin cancer. There would be a new team of support: two oncologists, nurse practitioners, nurses, melanoma specialty department head coordinators, surgeons, radiologists, pathologists, residents, orderlies, lab techs, lymphedema specialists, and all other staff members who will make your upcoming hospital visit most enjoyable. My head was trying to keep it all organized but was reeling for sure.

I should have known He would be here in the middle of all my fear. As I was driving, I noticed I was getting upset, overwhelmed, and agitated. Was it with my God whom I was agitated with? As I was praying on my way to my appointment, I felt the frustration of all my burdens and said out loud in the car, "Why am I even talking? You already know all my thoughts, all my worries, and how all this will play out and my feeling ... that I can't take one - more - thing - on my plate. You already know! So I am going to stop talking. See, I am not talking." I stopped talking. My eyes welled with tears. I kept thinking, *He knows, He already knows. He knows everything.* I took some deep breaths, slowly, like I had taught many of my patients in the past when they would have an anxious moment. Deeply breathe in through the nose, and with pursed lips out through the mouth slowly, exhaling to count of eight. I did this a few more times. So this is what feeling overwhelmed is like. There was nothing but silence in my car and the sound of my own breathing. Then I turned on my radio and fiddled with the dial to switch stations to "The Message," the Christian music station. The first four words that played from the radio were 'He knows, He knows.' The song is by Jeremy Camp. A great song and it was mid chorus. I had heard it once before. It was as if the Holy Spirit were saying, *He is hearing you, Lita. He knows what you have been through, and He knows what you can handle. He will give you enough strength to do so, trust me.*

The timing? This spot-on timing is God's perfect timing. For my ears needed to hear this, to calm my racing heart and thoughts. It was this exact moment on probably one of the most overwhelming days of my life that I felt alone, and my life seemed like it was out of control. I could not believe I was even needing an oncologist. And just minutes before my doctor's visit with everything on my plate, He made His Presence known. I had felt His Presence. Having arrived in the parking lot, I put my head on my steering wheel and, within the quiet moment in my car, I whispered: "Thank you."

The Holy Spirit just paid me a visit, I told myself. *Do not forget this drive today, for you certainly have someone listening in and hearing you!* His Omnipresence and perfect timing, wow! That is when I realized my strength comes from the Holy Spirit. He helps our Lord with His work here on earth all day long, every single day. Am I listening enough? I have stopped using the word "coincidence." Nope, no coincidence here today. This was certainly a Holy-Spirit moment. He knows, He knows.

CHAPTER SEVEN

IN THE BEGINNING

HISTORY OF THE BIBLE

When I began doing research, while interesting for sure, it became quite an overwhelming process to grasp the scope and depth of how the compilation of the Bible came to be. The Bible is a unified book of both the Old and New Testaments. The Old Testament is the record of God's creation. It gives us Laws to live by and prophesies the coming of the Messiah or Savior for all the world. The New Testament is the documentations of a 'fulfilled' prophecy as outlined in the Old Testament in which Jesus, the promised Savior, while on this earth, teaches us how to fulfill the laws and commandments in which we are to live by while commanding us to proclaim the Kingdom of Heaven. Upon His death, Jesus Christ epitomized *Grace and Mercy* for redemption to be received at any time by anyone through His death on the cross. He centers us with the Holy Spirit once He defeated the grave so we would not feel alone. God reveals himself in the Trinity—with God the Father, Jesus His Son, and the Holy Spirit. The body of believers to be forever One in Christ.

But for the purpose of this 'baby step' book, the complexities of how to adequately and truthfully display it here, well, I could not do it the justice it deserves. This is an area that should be left to the experts—truly. Multiple timelines exist chronologically displaying the Old Testament biblical documentation of its Law, History, Prophecy and Wisdom as Creation came into existence and the events of the world unfolded before the birth of Jesus Christ. The New Testament is twenty-seven books of printed scriptures representing the updated covenant revealed by Christ, with the earliest texts or letters dating back to AD 50–62. However, the discovery of the Dead Sea Scrolls in 1946 was the proof that gave weight and substantiated the writings of the Bible. It is irrefutable. It is not hard to research things these days as there is no need for encyclopedias anymore. It is so interesting to discover new things and one can certainly explore this further; it is literally at our fingertips with the internet. So after reading from various sites online and digging in a little deeper, what remained consistent in regards to the Dead Sea Scrolls was the following:

The Dead Sea Scrolls are a collection of 800–900 documents, many containing ancient sacred biblical texts. Some are in fragments of parchment and papyrus totaling over 50,000 individual pieces. Others are substantial and complete, the longest scroll being eight meters long. They were discovered in a series of almost one dozen caves around the site known as Wadi Qumran near the Dead Sea in the West Bank of the Jordan River between 1946 and 1956 by a team of archeologists and Bedouin shepherds. They were thought to be written by ancient Jewish sect called the Essenes. There continues to be a debate by scholars as to how far back they actually date. Some scholars say between 150 BC and AD 57. The only complete book of the Hebrew Bible preserved among the manuscripts from Qumran is Isaiah. This copy dated to the first century BC is considered the earliest Old Testament manuscript still in existence. They are thought to include fragments of every book of the Old Testament except for the Book of Esther.

The Bible is without parallel in its popularity or writing success that has continued influencing generations of people through the ages and spans the globe far and wide. And it will continue to have a profound impact for centuries to come. What I have discovered within my spiritual journey as raw emotions surfaced was every time I wanted to look up what the Bible had to say about a certain emotion, it was there. I found it could cover the width and breadth of every humanly possible emotion or feeling. It covers it all and in detail. Certainly we can always find books on love and respect, anxiety and depression, pain, fear, loss and sorrow, etc. The Bible addressed all of these feelings and provided me with encouragement, understanding, healing, and hope when I needed it most. We the people of here and now, those who have come before us, and those who will come after us will certainly experience a realm of emotions during the trials of this life. God already knew this and provided us with a tool or way to understand these emotions, with Him as our Tutor.

So as the galaxies were formed and our world evolved to include the existence of man, however you believe it occurred, this is where science and Christianity can be found to coexist. Have you ever given a second thought to all the factors that have to line up perfectly in order for life to exist at all on this planet we call Earth? The exact distance from the sun, its gravitational pull, rotation, and atmospheric pressure? The vision of all creation coming to fruition at the hand of my Lord I consider to be the first miracle. For He made sure there would be chosen ones to begin the documentation or prophesy as found in the Dead Sea scrolls, long before He would send the world a Savior, Jesus, to walk the earth. As the centuries unfolded this influentially profound writing continued, until we had 'One Book.' A unified book that will forever remain pertinent. There is no other book that has demonstrated to have such a worldly impact or power on humankind as this One Book—the Word. His Word. Whether you have read it or not, the BIBLE has and will continue to change the world. Forever.

In all the baby steps I have taken as I have journeyed through this course for my spiritual and physical well-being, I am beginning to notice a relationship forming as I understand more about what it means to know my Supreme Father. It is still overwhelming to me, and I feel so small when I remember this is a God who was not created but already existed.

WHAT IS FAITH?

Faith is believing in a Promise that cannot be seen. It is a sense of quiet confidence and public conviction of an eternal spiritual truth. It is a chosen and welcomed gift which is invisible, has no taste, texture, or aroma, and must reside in the impenetrable depths of one's soul. To have faith in the Trinity—God the Father, Jesus Christ, His only begotten Son, and the Holy Spirit—is a concept of truths that goes beyond the limits of understanding and requires complete, unquestionable and independent acceptance with belief. Faith is a gift waiting for you to unwrap it, allowing your heart to feel the presence of Christ residing within it, and securing your place in heaven.

I thought of how to try and explain the Trinity in a unique and memorable way, as the concept can be confusing for old and new believers. As this book is twofold and I have referred to lymph nodes in parts of this book as 'pearls,' it came to me as I thought of a beautiful strand of pearls. Some of the rarest strands of high-quality saltwater pearls are worth millions of dollars. According to Wikipedia, the 'La Peregrina Pearl' is probably the most famous pearl in the world. It is said that for every 10,000 oysters harvested, only one will contain a 'high-quality' pearl. The scarcity of natural pearls in turn make them extremely valuable. They are sought after by the rich and famous, royal families, celebrities, and jewelry connoisseurs from all over the world. They will spend millions of dollars to get their hands on high-quality saltwater pearls.

So as I think of the Trinity and what the pearl symbolizes: wisdom, purity, generosity, integrity, and loyalty; when it is worn, I see similarities. First, our God possesses all these character traits and more. A pearl emerges and is formed around a *single grain of sand* within the mollusks, as it tries to protect itself by coating this irritant with calcium carbonate, which is salt found in nature. From a single grain of sand, a pure, rare and valuable gemstone can be formed.

THE HOLY TRINITY

The Trinity symbolizes three in one, or one God in three persons. A strand of pearls in its creation—with the clasp or box, hook, and silk threading—symbolizes the Trinity. Once the necklace is graced with the addition of each pearl, the unity of the strand with the embodiment of believers make it one exquisite and priceless piece.

The first and main part of the strand is *the clasp or box*, whose placement around the neck can be worn to be seen in any position. This clasp symbolizes Our God the Father. It is usually very opulent, encrusted with diamonds and gemstones, and can make a statement all on its own. At the same time, the clasp can be visually understated, so the pearls and the entire strand can be appreciated. This is the heavyweight, with a unique shape. Within its boxlike shape clasp is a small opening on one side to connect with a hook for closure of the strand. The clasp provides the foundation and stabilizes the strand around the neck. It is where the strand begins and where it ends, like the Alpha and Omega. The entire strand is dependent upon the clasp. If there was no clasp, the strand would not exist at all. This is Our God the Father, the key to our very existence.

The second part of the strand of pearls is *the hook*. Once the clasp or box is made, the hook is made for a perfect fit. It is immediately a safeguard 'unit' to expand upon. The Word, Jesus Christ, was with God since the beginning. The hook is usually in the shape of a 'V,' for Victory, in defeating death. It has a double safety factor in that with one tip of the 'V' is first hooked around a small bar in the opening of the boxlike clasp and then it is depressed further to slide into the opening on the clasp and snaps into place. This symbolizes the Son of God, Jesus Christ. This is the security for the strand to stay fastened while being worn. Through Jesus Christ, you secure your place in heaven. The hook is only valuable as its key function is to stay interlocked and connected to the clasp. Just as Jesus is always connected with the Almighty Father. When the two are linked, they become one unit and are even more powerful and stronger than you can imagine. It is only through Jesus that you can get to the Father through the forgiveness of sin. In perfect purity can we be before the throne. Without the hook, there could be no connection to secure to the clasp, and hence no strand.

The third part of the strand that symbolizes the Holy Spirit is the finely woven *thread of silk* that is first tied to the hook and ends being tied to the clasp. This silk thread is gently drawn through the center of each pearl, to be knotted on both sides of the pearl for added safety. Should anything happen to dislodge the entire strand, the pearls would not be lost. Once a part of the strand, always a part of the strand. This silk is a very strong fiber and is responsible for being centered in the pearl to keep it connected to the rest of the strand. The Holy Spirit is Jesus' gift to us, after He defeated the grave and ascended into heaven. Jesus works through the Holy Spirit here on earth. Which makes the Holy Spirit moments very real as they are centered within us. If there was no silk thread, there would be no strand.

The necklace becomes complete as *the pearls* themselves are added one by one. Which to me symbolizes the vision of our Creator from the beginning of time: it is man. The pearls—which are all unique, come in varying shapes and sizes with varying degree of luster—make up the strand. Their individual worth, beauty, and rarity is the reason to wear the strand in the first place. Each pearl is highly sought after and precious to the entire strand. But the pearls are so much more beautiful in a strand all together than as a single unit. And as they sit side by side on the strand, each pearl helps to accentuate the next. The pearl necklace in all its grandeur embodies the fellowship of believers as joined together by the Trinity. They can be connected directly to the Father, through the silk threading of the Holy Spirit and the security of the Promise through Jesus Christ who holds the direct link to God the Father, the clasp. If even one portion to this strand of pearls is missing, there would be no purpose for its existence at all. Hence, the sole purpose of the existence of this exquisite strand of pearls lies within its beauty and promise as a whole, and it can be an infinite length.

The La Peregrina Pearl

For a little jewelry history lesson, there have been many well-documented and luxurious strands of pearls. The top ten most valuable strands ranged in price from 1.6 to 7.1 million dollars. Their history and previous owners did play a role in their purchase price. But the La Peregrina Pearl was considered the most famous in the world. It was found in the mid-sixteenth century by an African slave off the coast of Santa Margarita, a Spanish colony in the Gulf of Panama. This rare discovery bought his freedom. It has a 500-year history being passed from royal to royal. Philip II, King of Spain, gifted it to Mary I, daughter of King Henry VIII and first wife Catherine of Aragon and Queen of England. And upon Mary I's death, it was returned to the crown of Spain and remained there for over 250 years. As it continued to change hands through the years, James Hamilton, fifth duke of Abercorn, had possessed it since 1870. But in 1969, Hamilton's estate sold it to Sotheby's auction in London, wherein actor Richard Burton was the highest bidder and purchased the infamous pearl for $37,000.00. Burton purchased it for his jewelry connoisseur and celebrity wife, Elizabeth Taylor, giving it to her as a gift on Valentine's Day. She had commissioned Cartier to reset the drop pearl with additional strands of pearls, and included other gems of diamonds and rubies. When some of her jewelry estate was auctioned off posthumously in 2011 by Christie's auctioneers, the La Peregrina pearl strand alone fetched an estimated $11,000,000.00 by a buyer in Asia. While the estimated value was slightly over $3,000,000.00, the fact it had such a significant history behind it is what made it extremely valuable.

CHAPTER EIGHT

ALWAYS SOMETHING TO THINK ABOUT

MORE OPTIONS TO CONSIDER

With my diagnosis of malignant melanoma cancer and micrometasta-sis, many appointments followed that included 'options' for the next steps. The options were much more difficult this go around. The risks were going to be higher, but incurring the risk may have its benefits of a thera-peutic outcome (I may end up cancer free). And again I would hear, "Either option is reasonable." At times I thought, *Am I taking this too seriously? Is it really not that bad? If either option was reasonable, then can I wait this out?*

I met with the melanoma clinic dermatology director, where she reviewed the latest statistics with the diagnosis I had. The survival rate is eighty percent after five years. She explained in detail how the diagnosis of staging was made and confirmed, and where my diagnosis fell compared to the more advanced stage IV's. I was stage III-A. Then she reviewed the potential outcomes for the options to choose from. The oncologist came in right after and discussed adjuvant therapy with me and all the associated risks. **Adjuvant therapy is medication that revs your immune system to promote its function.** They also informed me of a drug trial going on at Stanford which I would be a candidate for, and the trial counselor came in and very briefly summarized the trial. She gave me a copy of the trial consent to read at home, all twenty-eight pages of it. I was to call her for an appointment to review the consent in more detail should I decide to include this route.

The options given to me were reviewed as follows:

Option ONE: No more surgery and manage this with aggressive surveillance/diagnostic monitoring by use of ultrasound on the remaining lymph nodes every three months for three years. If there is something that shows up in the lymph area, or I palpate something new in the area, then a further discussion and a new plan will be made.

Option TWO: I can undergo a complete axillary lymph node dissection surgery. Meaning surgically remove the remaining axillary lymph nodes (pearls). This is around twenty-five to thirty of them and the procedure will take about three to four hours. This would aid in gaining knowledge if the cancer has invaded any other lymph nodes and possibly spread to other areas of the body. The risks associated with this kind of surgery are now escalated, as the immune system has been impacted to a greater degree once these will have been removed. The potential post-op complications are higher.

Option THREE: Start adjuvant therapy, which means additional medication by infusion and/or injection. This medication would be started within a reasonable amount of time. I had two weeks to think about it. I think immunotherapy is the 'happy' word for chemotherapy. People do not know what immunotherapy is. But it is called this because the medications used are supposed to boost your 'immune' system. It can also wreak havoc on your immune system, as that is the biggest risk factor associated with its treatment. This would be started after option one or option two was completed. Treatment would be for a few years. The risks associated with this treatment are very complicated and most definitely may change my life as I know it. I will discuss these risks very briefly later.

(Addendum: as of 1/2018, immunotherapy is now not even offered as a form of supportive (adjuvant) treatment for patients with stage IIIA melanoma, as the benefits associated with the medication do not outweigh the risks with it. New guidelines will be established to support the change, but the treatment options for any diagnosis will always be between the patient and physicians, including immunotherapy.)

Option FOUR: A clinical trial at Stanford hospital that has a promising 'arm.' 'Arms' are patient treatment groups which are studied comparing therapeutic outcomes of the medications given. In this case, two medications would be compared against each other, hence two arms, or patient treatment groups in the trial. They would be randomly selected and administered to qualified candidates from all over the country. They would be randomly assigned in a sequential order. I would be assigned and administered one of them. I would not know which medication I was assigned until I enrolled and was approved to be in the trial. There was no placebo to be used. There was a window of time in which you must enroll. BUT first, I would have to complete option TWO, which is removal of all remaining lymph nodes (my pearls). I would have to undergo the surgery and incur the associated risks of the surgery and undergo trial start by the 'window' of time. Your life is followed for a period of years, and a commitment to do random lab testing etc. would be outlined in a contract to be signed at enrollment. A brief discussion of the trial detail will be discussed later.

CHAPTER NINE

IS HE NEAR

HELPLESS IN FEAR - HE IS NEAR?

When I experienced fear, the emotional turmoil unleashed would usually occur in the days and weeks of 'waiting for something.' It most certainly manifested itself in a variety of ways—anxiety, worry, feeling of being helpless, fatigue, hopeless and loneliness—to name a few that would come and go for me. The reality is an emotion can be changed, but this is always easier said than done. It takes courage, desire, and strength, but it needs to be driven by 'choice.' All can usually come from within when we don't feel so broken. Many people will suffer a lifetime in these states and never seek out proper help. If not properly managed, spiraling into a darker world may occur over time. Often the daily strength it takes to keep the 'worry' away can be depleting and fatiguing in itself. The fear of what lies ahead is real and is occupying more of my thoughts than I like. I suppose it is normal. But one emotion seemed to lead to another. While I never allowed myself to wallow too long, I needed to understand how I could replenish my emotional wellbeing. Then I could focus on substituting my new learned behavior of daily quiet time 'whenever' I felt the need. My 'Bible' baby steps would become my focus.

Spiritual Pearl ~ Three

After months spending time in the morning hours reading and learning, I noticed I was starting to build an arsenal of great scripture quotes that I would refer to anytime. For if you have nothing to lean on, then you have NOTHING to lean on. This was my new 'something,' which would remind me of His Promise to me in so many different ways. He is here with me in times of fear. He is near, He hears me and knows my struggle, and He has me by my right hand. I leaned on this daily as I would wait for what awaited me. I was not disappointed in the comfort it provided me every single day.

This made it easier for me to control these untoward emotions from seeping in on me. What many do not understand is why it is so important to reenergize, nourish, or replenish what has otherwise been exhausted and depleted through our emotional turmoil. We need to refill our cups, to help maintain emotional wellness. I am thankful I have never experienced the depth that I know an emotion of darkness can dive into if we do not have something to help us replenish. I have seen it, counselled and treated many who have suffered with this. I have seen people reach for the wrong vice, alcohol, drugs (and they don't have to be illegal to be misused) thinking this will help—it never does, and the abyss gets deeper. I will choose to fuel my soul, exactly how I am telling you I did. This was the only way to restore the balance I usually have. We can be replenished easily by our Limitless Giver. We need to find that 'Trust' to provide the 'Hope' that then provides the 'Strength' to move forward day after day. Otherwise, we will *feel* defeated and we will *be* defeated.

> *"Never be afraid to trust an unknown future to a known God."*
>
> (CORRIE TEN BOOM)

I don't take credit for this great line. I heard it in a song, but cannot remember the artist. I am sorry. As I continued to read my handful of books, switching off here and there, I came across another journal entry and I would read this over and over.

'When we no longer feel like we can manipulate our circumstance in our favor is when fear can set in. This is when we need to say," Lord, my Father, this is out of my control. I need you because I am afraid. I might feel helpless, but there is no need for me to feel 'hopeless.'" I find comfort in anticipating how God will miraculously intervene in my circumstances. He will always have the best for those who wait for Him and are obedient to Him. Doing what is right. I will not allow my emotions to have free reign, nor will I be at the mercy of fear. I have just experienced the joy that comes in knowing He heard me. He was listening ... to me.'

Some of you reading this may have a much bigger challenge ahead of you or behind you even than I have experienced to date. Such independent journeys for each of us. I would highly recommend the book I mentioned, *The Strength You Need.* Throughout each chapter, it immediately became relevant and helpful to me almost daily. Chapter after chapter I became engrossed in the wisdom and insight the author had. It was as if he were speaking directly to me. I needed to find the strength so as not to be consumed with fear. Fear of the unknown. Fear in the waiting days and nights ahead. Fear in how my life would be after this is over. Fear for my family coping with all that awaited ahead. I recommend journaling and taking notes: they are great references, and be sure you write down the scripture verse you quoted from. So here are a just a few of my favorite one-liners.

"Be still, and know that I am God."

PSALM 46:10

"The Lord will fight for you, you need only 'be still'."

EXODUS 14:14

"For I am the Lord your God, who takes you by the right hand and says to you, Do Not Fear, I Will Help You."

ISAIAH 41:13

Walking close side by side so He can empower me to face the daily tasks ahead with a grateful heart is my course. So much encouragement as I keep reading, and such great writing by experienced authors. I am like a sponge absorbing this up. The more I try to learn in strengthening my faith, and the more I spend time in the Word, the more I recognize 'trust' is slowly replacing my fear. I can trust Him and I will place my trust in Him. After all, trust is what is missing when fear is all-consuming, especially with fear of the unknown. This is something I noticed took practice for me: I would see the human part of me allow it to creep back in on occasion, especially in the guts of the challenge. I find if I engage in conversation with Him and be still trying to listen to His answer, I can imagine what He might be saying to me. It takes practice and I don't know if I am totally there at times. But I did not stop engaging with Him. I still have no idea what awaits me.

This book called the Bible is so rich for my soul. Its food for my mind and body. But sometimes I am relying on myself a bit too much. I mean that I have been doing this all my life. Now relinquishing all control, well, it is all I can do. I am positive He can do a better job than I could ever do.

MY FIRST SWIM - A VISION FROM THE HEAVENS

With another upcoming appointment very near after the options have been reviewed, the time has come to finalize in greater detail which sequence of options I would prefer. The goal for this appointment is to have all my questions answered, address any last-minute concerns, and decide the immediate next steps. I would meet with my cutaneous oncology surgeon once again, and then my oncologist would discuss the possibility regarding immunotherapy and the trial available for my stage III A. I would be able to get my surgery on her books.

I have not been able to work out, aside from a walk here or there for a couple of months, as I had pneumonia prior to my last surgery. I knew that another surgery most likely was in my near future, and that would set my swimming workout back even further. The incurred risks associated with a complete axillary lymph node dissection remain unknown. I do not know what my future post-op course would bring, nor if I would ever swim again. The risks and potential complications for any surgery is real and should be considered. I am one of those people who prefer to understand the details and not take the ignorance-is-bliss approach.

My doctor had given me the all-clear to go swimming once my wounds were healed. After all, there was almost a five-inch incision on my scapular area and about a four-inch incision under my left arm. Both had healed up nicely. I continued to have a sensation of something pulling in my upper back area, but suspected this was probably normal. She knew I was a swimmer and that it would be therapeutic for me to resume my activities. I have always swam as part of my workouts and have for years. Not that I am in great shape, but it is my preferred sport when I need to get a workout in. I found my body to have great muscle memory with swim activity. I love to swim laps: it is second nature to me. I especially love the feel of the water rushing over my body when I first dive in. The world silence that immediately follows when my head submerges underwater and the peace that follows each lap is sublime.

With each length of the pool, my thoughts focus on improving my stroke. I pay attention to my body and hip alignment, my hand entry, my kicking and breathing rhythm. I can choose to be in prayer while I am swimming, as there is no other distraction for me. Some of my most inspiring thoughts for this book came to me while I was swimming. Before I pray for anything, I thank Him for everything. Everything in my life is a gift from Him. I feel like a fish when I swim, like I belong. Weird I know, but I am sure my deep love for the ocean stems from the fact it is where I learned to swim. Swimming in a pool or the ocean is cathartic for me, providing such psychological cleansing. It was a talent He gave me and I excelled at it, so I grew to love it. When I swim, I'm not thinking about the laundry, bills, or even what we're having for dinner (though I could if I wanted to, but I don't), so I enjoy the moments I have in the pool. But at the same time, I can also choose to focus on something that may be bothering me. I can ponder over it while I am in the water and, usually between the two of us, can come up with an answer. I am in another world when I get to pay the water a visit. So I have no fear of it and I could not wait to get back to it!

I put my suit on the morning of April 4th and drove to the club. It was an early beautiful pristine spring morning, and fabulous central California weather. When I arrived to pick my lane, I noticed I had the entire pool to myself. I looked around and there was not a single person in sight who would be joining me in the water today, which usually never happens. I love swimming in a pool where the water is clean, blue, and perfectly still. Not even a single ripple could be seen. I thought to myself, and said, "Wow, Lord, did you do this for me? You know how much I have been looking forward to this swim, and you already know of my worry that I may never be able to swim again. Thank you for giving me this perfect day." So, with my cap and goggles on, I dove in.

All those feelings of how much I enjoy this sport flooded back as I glided through and underwater for nearly half the length of the pool. Next to the last lap of a tough workout, the first lap is simply the best. It felt so good. With my arms extended gently overhead, my body completely submerged, relaxed, and streamline, I felt halfway human again. I took it easier than usual and was pleased with my progress in the movement with my arm. I was appreciative of each stroke. Swimming is the best therapy for this type of surgery: you will hear me mention this more than once! How fortunate am I—it's what I love to do most.

Holy Spirit Moment ~ TWO

As I continued with my workout, I turned onto my back to swim some backstroke. When I looked up to the sky, I noticed a formation of large wispy clouds directly above me. And only above me. Intently I looked again, because I could not believe I was seeing what I was seeing.

The face of my sweet Jesus, peering down at me. I could see both eyes on His face perfectly outlined and they had a slight downward slant at the outer corners. The surprise was even the irises were visible within both eyes and were perfectly centered and round. Both of His brows were visible, the full length of His nose and then His beard and hair flowed and trailed off, both above and below His face. It was majestic, glorious, and gigantic in appearance. I was in awe. *Oh, my goodness!* I thought. Then with excitement I said, "You are watching over me and I see you!" There was no one else in the pool that I could say, "Hey, do you see what I see in that cloud formation up there?" Not a single person on deck was around to witness what I had just seen. It was for my eyes only. On my drive home, I called my husband to share what a perfect morning it had been, for I have seen the face of Jesus in the clouds within the heavens. Oh, my goodness.

When I got home, I showered and got ready to have my quiet time. He deserves much more attention than He receives from me. But this morning, I owe Him this and I must sit and listen. So after this perfect swim on this pristine morning, with my glorious vision everything became even clearer to the reality of His existence. I read from one of my daily devotionals and then looked up the biblical scripture associated with it and jotted down, on this memorable morning of April 4th, 2017, and it all fell into place.

"For the eyes of the Lord range throughout the earth to strengthen those whose hearts are fully committed to Him,"

2 CHRONICLES 16:9

"He makes me lie down in green pastures, He leads me beside quiet waters, He refreshes my soul. He guides me along the right paths for His name sake,"

PSALM 23:2–3

"Be still before the Lord, all mankind, because He has roused himself from His holy dwelling,"

ZECHARIAH 2:13

I see the significance in ALL three of these scriptures and how my amazing morning unfolded before my eyes. For on this day the scriptures revealed first that He was looking for me. Second, He met me in the stillness of the water, as I have been trying to give my whole heart to Him and He has nourished my soul. Third, He rose in the Heavens to pay me a visit.

I was excitedly anticipating and waiting to see what He planned to reveal next. He once again had my undivided attention. Might I remind you the writing of this book had not even been a mere thought for me as yet. Probably to Him, but not to me.

That weekend we were going to have a family meeting to discuss my surgery. I shared my vision in the clouds with my daughters and granddaughters. I drew the image I recalled so vividly upside down. And as my granddaughter watched me sketch this on paper, before the entire image even unfolded she said, "Gigi, that looks like Jesus. That is really good!" She is six years old. The truth of this vision may be more believable if you had seen it. I will never forget it, and I am beginning to pay more attention. My senses have been on high alert, if you will. Because for some reason, He is making His presence known to me. I am seeing it and hearing it more and more, and I am not quite sure why. No more coincidences here. Not to me. This is what I drew. I didn't ever want to forget this perfect first swim.

What do you see in the clouds? So then I gave 'one attempt' to paint a water color of my vision. The sky that day was a canvas of His Grace!

Can you even imagine?

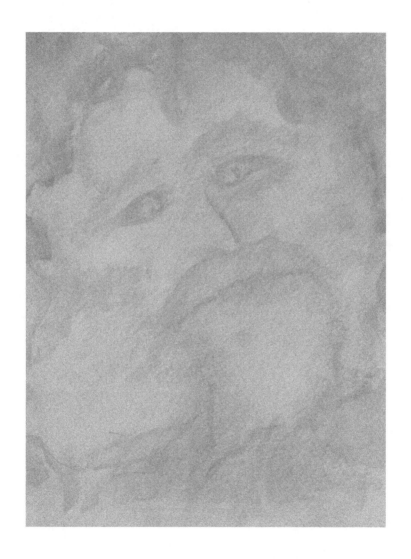

CHAPTER TEN

NOT TO BE TAKEN LIGHTLY

WEIGHING THE OPTIONS

My husband and I made the three-hour drive again—mostly because of commuter traffic—to visit all of our new friends at Stanford Medical Center, for a discussion that as I mentioned was to be more serious today. I was really looking forward to all of my team of doctors weighing in on what I should do. All of the options we had been mulling over since my one-week post-op visit after the first surgery. Today was decision time after two weeks of thinking about it.

Once again I get settled in the exam room and greetings were exchanged. I was able to share what a great swim I had with my surgeon and how thankful I was to have been able to do that. She was pleased with this progress. She did a quick examination of my prior wound, as this was the site she would reenter to do the completion surgery. I told her I was pretty sure I wanted to proceed with the complete axillary lymph node dissection surgery and as she spoke, in her soft and gentle voice she emphasized this surgery would be different. She wanted to make it perfectly clear that this next surgery, if I go through with it and all goes well, would present a much tougher recovery course. The pain would be intense and the risk of complications greater as there is more involved. She reminded me again she would do everything she could to identify and preserve the main nerves that support the arm. On the flip side, a therapeutic cure from this surgery would be welcomed and is the ultimate hope. If I can never swim again, it will have been worth it.

She began with the facts, and reviewed again that I have two options: first option is to do surveillance monitoring with every-three-month axillary ultrasounds for three years. If the melanoma cancer cells were going to spread, it would first show in the swelling of a node under my arm, causing a lump. They would monitor the size and if there were changes, then the next step would be discussed, which would be surgery. I got a little leery with this option; after all, I have been so diligent and proactive with all of my skin checks and follow-ups. Why would I slow this down now? The second option is to do the complete axillary lymph node dissection surgery. The adjuvant therapy and trial was to be discussed after this visit. She clarified it would be another three to three-and-a-half-hour surgery, under general anesthesia. I guess there was also a third option: to do absolutely nothing.

She explained the surgery in detail. Stated she would go in through the same incision I already have, except she would need to make the incision larger. I would have a suction drain that had a bulb on the end of it and it would be sutured into place in the outer skin area. The suction bulb's duty was to drain the typical postlymphatic fluid that would continue to flow and accumulate in the pocket she just created by removing what was previously there. The faucet is still running. The drainage would be red in appearance at first, but after a few days should change to the color of apple juice. I would need to keep track of the drainage by emptying the bulb twice daily. Most likely the drain would remain in place for a week or two. The drains are removed once the amount of fluid decreases in the bulb. The goal was to have less than twenty milliliters for two days in a row for the drains to come out. But the longer the drains remain in place, the increased risk of infection.

You see, once the lymph nodes are removed, the lymph drainage continues to flow until it recognizes it needs to reroute itself. This process can take a very long time. It is like if you left the hose running. The only way the water is going to stop is if you shut the main valve off. Well, there is no shutting the main valve off in your body. Sometimes the rerouting is a very slow process, hence swelling of the entire arm or part of the arm occurs. Pain medication would definitely be needed. This postsurgical recovery would be much more painful and more limiting. My drain would follow me wherever I would go, for who knows how long. I needed to keep my arm elevated as much as possible, and it would be difficult to lie on my left side. I wondered if I would be well enough to still make the trip to Maui that we had booked in January before all this started. It was scheduled for mid June.

She informed me that before I proceeded with surgery, I would need a test called the **L-Dex (lymphedema index) test. This is a measurement monitoring system used to aid in the clinical assessment of unilateral changes in cellular fluid, or lymphatic fluid of the arm.** This test, which takes about two seconds to complete, needs to be done prior to surgery to establish a baseline that would be considered 'my normal' and then repeated every three months. They would schedule them starting three months after the completion surgery and every three months thereafter for the first year. This allows the lymphedema specialists to evaluate if there is any unilateral cellular changes in the skin due to the increased lymphatic drainage that has nowhere to go. Hence the swelling starts. The earlier the swelling from abnormal cellular fluid change is caught, the sooner it can be minimized. The swelling can be very painful and be immobilizing, making it difficult to bend at the elbow or wrist or even shoulder. In some cases, wearing a full arm sleeve would be advisable. In fact all undergoing this type of surgery should at least be measured for a proper sleeve fitting by a certified lymphedema therapist, and have one on hand in case it is needed.

I was given a list of all that was involved, including the most worrisome risk of a twenty percent chance of infection and loss of the use of my arm. Two major nerves could possibly be severed during this more complicated surgery. But these nerves can be exposed, identified, and protected. Without getting technical, they affect your posture and the ability to raise your shoulders, or lift an arm.

My cutaneous oncology surgeon was confident in her surgical skills, and promised that once again it would be her job to identify and protect those nerves. I asked her, if I were her sister, what would she have me do? I do think a physician should have an opinion. But what I have come to appreciate is that they take into consideration what your life is already like. Are you a busy, active, on-the-go person, or do you have more of a sedentary, quieter lifestyle? Does this option or that option work best for you? It is my life that will be effected, not theirs. Therefore, it would need to be my decision, and she stated either option is reasonable. Whether I do surveillance monitoring or the surgery, my survival rate would be the same. Either route would still carry an eighty percent survival rate in five years. Meaning, one option has not proved to be the 'better' of the two options regarding a survival outcome.

That is all well and good, but for me anyway my thinking is if I can give my physicians more diagnostic information with this dissection of more nodes, and information is knowledge for an optimum plan, and surgery may be a therapeutic cure … hmmm. I feel there is a peace of mind in one of these options, but it takes on a very big associated risk factor. The other option is a wait and wait to see if you have any node size changes, then a plan is formulated. Both will impact your life in some facet. I have to decide.

I spent the next hour-and-a-half talking to my oncologist regarding adjuvant treatment, which is offered as comanagement treatment with Stage III-A. Discussion in brief of the trial that Stanford had going on for my diagnosis qualified me as a potential candidate. The risks regarding immunotherapy were reviewed in an overwhelming fashion. I was trying so hard to remember the risk of a GI bleed, ulcerative colitis, and adrenal failure, and risk of parathyroid gland shutdown. Extreme fatigue, diarrhea, rash, nausea, headache, and possible weight loss would be a normal encounter. The weight loss was the only thing that sounded good to me! Seriously, I am no expert to discuss in detail all the risks associated with adjuvant therapy, but it sounded awful and, quite frankly, I was scared to death. I once again could not believe I was having a discussion like this and that this was even being recommended. Of course it would be up to me, again it would be my decision. The benefit of doing the immunotherapy (remember it is medication to help boost your immune system, rev it up so to speak) would improve my survival rate by six to seven percent. Wait, what? Did I hear that correctly? So I repeated it back and yes, I had heard it correctly.

I then met with the immunotherapy trial counselor again, and she very briefly (an hour) reviewed a twenty-eight-page document with me. She told me to take it home and read it thoroughly but not sign it. If I was interested in the trial, I was to make an appointment back with her for complete consent review and signature. That appointment would take about an hour and a half. If I were to be in the trial, then I must have the completion surgery done. The trial would usually start within six to eight weeks after the surgery. I would start the trial medication arm I had been assigned. Okay, I got it. I was to call with my decision within the next one or two weeks. If surgery was the avenue we chose, she would get me on her schedule as soon as it permitted. In the meantime while I am deciding, I will need to have a PET (positron emission tomography) scan and brain MRI (magnetic resonance imaging) since I tested positive for melanoma cancer cells in the lymph nodes. Those tests were being ordered, so I would be awaiting a call from radiology.

The minute we got in the car, I said to my husband, "Did you get all that?" My husband grasped more than I thought he would. He said, "Why would anyone do the immunotherapy? The chance of something happening is greater than the benefit it provides!" I was like, *Wow, you do get it.* Most of us providers would always give our patients the benefits and risks of a particular medication or treatment option. Does the benefit of taking the medication outweigh the risks associated with the medication? I just could not feel it in this case. I get nauseated just thinking about having to do the immunotherapy.

Now, the trial had possibilities, as one of the arms was a drug, Pembrolizumab (Keytruda), which is proving to be promising. It is already being used for Stage IV melanoma, and they are trying to get it approved for Stage III-A, which is why there is a trial at all. They want to compare the effects, good or bad, of the experimental drug, Keytruda, to the usual treatment of interferon alfa-2b or ipilimumab (IPI).

Keytruda is indicated as treatment for patients with unresectable or metastatic melanoma. It had a better increase for survival rate by up to thirty to forty percent. Sounded like we need to read the consent and have further discussion on this one. But this was not a guarantee that I would be given this medication in the trial. But the other arm of the trial uses two choices for an immunotherapy drug that I would get to choose from. One is the interferon, and the other is ipilimumab (IPI or Yervoy). I am not going to get into the medication; it is too much to cover and super frightening to read about. You can google it.

So the risks had all been reviewed in detail. I really appreciated their patience with me. I was trying to keep all the statistics straight in my mind. Because in the end, you want to make a decision where the benefit of that decision does outweigh any looming risks without it. I have heard doctors say that melanoma is such a 'ghost' of a cancer when one cell goes rogue, and it can also be a real monster.

FIRST FAMILY MEETING

Now we were going to have a family meeting regarding what my next steps of treatment would involve the following afternoon. My daughters and their husbands would come for dinner. The discussion would include the possible complications of the completion of axillary lymph node dissection, as well as reviewing the side effects from the adjuvant therapy and the medication arms of being in the trial, which we had not done before. This would allow them to clearly understand and ask any questions should they have any concerns, and saved me from repeating myself six times. I am a firm believer that information is knowledge and knowledge is key for an informed decision. Again, some people may want to take the ignorance-is-bliss route. I get why, but I just cannot do it.

Their thoughts were very important to my husband and me. This next step, especially if surgery and immunotherapy are a part of it, will impact the entire family. I may really need some help, and that burden they wanted to fall on them. They got a vote. My daughters are at an age where they wanted to be encouraging, helpful, and supportive. They had made a pact with each other that they would divulge to me later. I would never have to go to the doctor alone. So precious of them, but unrealistic as they are busy mothers and wives too. The promise we had made to each other, of being transparent when any one of us was going through something difficult, needed to be kept also. I had promised to be honest with them on how I was feeling on any particular day. They knew that if I fell silent for a couple of days, I might be struggling with pain or worry. I felt they deserved to be included and have a choice in the plan, as well as my sons-in-law. I know their personalities and how much they each worry about things. Plus they really needed to understand the potential impact.

We said a prayer before dinner, asking for a clear picture of what option would prove to be the most promising. The dishes were cleared and we all sat at the dining room table to discuss this looming shadow. I began by reviewing the options that I have already shared with you. I said it was important to me that they really understand the impact the surgery may have on me, what immunotherapy was, and what the trial meds are all about. My biggest fear, I told them, was recalling two friends who have had their own battle with malignant melanoma stage III-A, with such difficult treks for both. One of them lost their battle after two years of immunotherapy, with extremely difficult GI issues and metastasis. The other had lymphedema of the lower extremity with complete adrenal failure and parathyroid gland dysfunction after several infusions of immunotherapy. Neither gave me any hope.

I began with some of the verbiage stated in the twenty-eight-page consent form. Seriously. I started reading the risks associated with the meds, and right away I said, "I will not do interferon alpha 2-b, so that is out." That leaves me with IPI, or I can hope I get the arm in the trial of Keytruda. There is no guarantee that I would be assigned this drug. But if I did not get the arm I preferred, I could opt out. You were not bound to do the trial; only if you started in the trial would you be required to complete it.

I went through the associated risks in a little more detail. Then on to the surgery risks. I explained it to them just as I have explained it to you. The impact on the immune system I have shared with you. My immune system will be compromised forever, so I must refrain from exposure to illnesses. Meaning be careful when around people who are ill, including sick grandchildren. My job was also to protect my arm from any form of injury, right down to trying to prevent a mosquito bite. With this surgery, it is so important to be careful with any type of bites. Sunburns are a no-no, and protecting your skin from cracking is important too. I would need to really protect my arm after surgery and forever more. There would also be physical limitations. I couldn't lift anything for a while, not even my new grandson who would be five months old. And no pulling or pushing anything until given the all-clear.

You may be thinking why review all this with everyone in such detail since it is my decision. But the reality was a twenty percent chance I may suffer from something that would require help, temporarily, needed to be understood. Twenty percent may not sound very high to you, but in the medical world it is. My family is the type that prefers to know what is going on. If there was a complication, it would help being informed and prepared for this. Now this does not mean I am being pessimistic; it means I am being cautious and real. It means my life as I know it may take a turn. Until I figured out how to accomplish certain daily routines, as even paraplegics learn to adjust, I would need assistance until I could adjust and find my new normal.

It seriously crossed my mind: what if I cannot use my left arm? I would need help doing things I am not even aware of and definitely take for granted. Stupid things too, like, how do I close my car door, being this is on my left side, how would I put my hair in a ponytail? How do you fold clothes, or lift something up off the ground? Put a necklace on, tie my shoes? You get the picture. Then there would be no more sports activities, like swimming laps, no tennis matches, as I wouldn't be able to serve the ball, no snow skiing. And the toughest one: I cannot babysit, because I could not lift my grandson out of his crib. Someone can place him in my lap when I am sitting down, but no more picking him up. Sometimes I wonder if we providers really think about all these things for our patient. But in the end getting rid of the cancer is the number one goal, and we just have to take one day at a time. I've always been one to see and evaluate a broader picture.

I know I would adjust in time; it is who I am. It may take me some time, but I will get there. However, this is a leery choice. Where is my Faith? Where is my Trust? I was feeling I could trust my surgeon to do her best. But as I once again relinquish control in this circumstance and find I am at the mercy of what I believe to be skilled hands, I have to wonder, where should have I placed my trust and faith? Surely God will not let this happen. But I seem to be relying on her expertise when I should have been thanking Him for what He is about to do. He can certainly intervene any time if He wishes. And in any situation He can change it. But what if He doesn't? Sometimes things don't always work out like we'd hoped they would. How will I really feel then about everything? I won't know until it happens. What will my Chief of Staff decide to do with me?

Immunotherapy—is it for me? We continue to discuss immunotherapy (interferon or IPI): there is a twenty percent chance of increased risk of infection, diarrhea, nausea, vomiting, flulike symptoms, aches, muscle pain, fatigue, appetite loss, weight loss, anemia, headache, depression or thoughts of suicide, hair loss, fever, and chills—to name a few. The more serious risks that carry a four-to-twenty percent chance would include heart failure, abnormal heartbeat, low blood pressure, blood clots, diabetes, bruising, damage to organs, stroke, coma, blurred vision, etc. You can pretty much count on experiencing tiredness, diarrhea, and nausea. The diarrhea may be a result of intestinal problems (colitis) that can lead to tears or holes in the intestine. It also may attack your immune system and cause itching, rash, blisters in the mouth, and hives. Possible kidney problems, liver problems, and hormonal gland problems are a risk. Goodness.

So I continue reading, and with all eyes looking at me. Initially when we discussed the possibility of a medication, we all thought maybe this would be a good idea, for an added proactive measure. I was encouraged to con- sider immunotherapy in the trial, but all these risks should not be taken lightly. I noticed when I was going through these risks I mentioned above, the paper in my hand started shaking, and I couldn't read things very clear. Then I realized it was because my hands were trembling and my eyes were filling with tears. I am telling you this part of the decision-making process really troubled me to the core. My husband asked me why I was crying. I thought for what seemed like a long pause and said; "Because my biggest fear is that my personality is going to change." Silly, right? This held a higher probability than the medication providing me additional protection. I like me, and the 'me' that they know may struggle while on this immune-boost- ing medication. My two friends who battled with melanoma experienced adrenal and parathyroid gland failure. Thyroid medication and other medications to counteract other symptomology became a part of their health care plan.

I believe in appropriate medicinal management for most of the issues that can arise from the risks, but I was worried the most about this. Would I be functioning in a strong happy mental place? I have no vices to try and sustain a mood or create a mood for that matter. The side effect potential would be out of my control. Yikes. I knew at this time I did not want to rely on more medication to correct whatever complication the immunotherapy medication could potentially cause. Did you get that? I do believe medication has its proper place with illnesses, and we have come a long way with new drug therapies. But I don't need any of them right now, and I am happy. God within me has made me 'who' I am. If this is a gut reaction, is God telling me something?

After about a thirty-five-minute discussion, the conclusion was: I did not think I could do the immunotherapy, period. I guess it became clearer to me, as I realized why I was so bothered with the thought of this. So adjuvant therapy for me was not going to be an option. Well, just when I thought we made a decision, we waffled back and forth, and waffled some more over these options for the next week. Sometimes I would change my mind two to three times per day: surgery then the trial, no surgery or immunotherapy just scans, okay just immunotherapy—no surgery and no trial, okay, okay, okay, wait I got it … surgery only. We prayed and prayed for clarity. Oh God, please make it clear to me. Then it came: why would I change and do the 'wait and watch' approach when I have been so proactive up until now? No matter the risk associated with this invasive surgery. After all, being proactive was the reason this had been caught early in the first place. There is my answer: I have to do this.

CHAPTER ELEVEN

LIFE MAY CHANGE

SURGERY IS THE PLAN

So it was decided and I let everyone know: I was going to do the complete axillary lymph node dissection surgery and 'consider' the trial. The reality: I was not sure I wanted to do any form of immunotherapy, in the trial or otherwise. Plus the trial was at Stanford, and that would be where I would have to travel to take part. That alone was going to be fatiguing. I remain confident with my decision and felt more diagnostic information available meant knowledge for my physicians and a better understanding of my prognosis. And as mentioned, it might be a therapeutic cure. That just means it may be a form of treatment on its own. If this next surgery proves to be negative for anymore melanoma cancer cells found in the excised remaining lymph nodes, I may be cured. Therapeutic, as now this proves all the melanoma cancer cells had been excised with the initial SLN biopsy. I will stay the course.

After four weeks of serious deliberation, the surgeon wanted to see me at the end of March and be sure this is what I wanted. This visit gave me an opportunity to get a second opinion regarding my right breast abscess, as this has not been resolved. It had been improving, but was still painful and present. If this abscess needed to be drained again, doing it with this upcoming surgery, if possible, would be appreciated. This will be the third time I will have undergone general anesthesia in less than five months. I was trying to prevent a fourth general anesthesia. I discussed this issue with my surgeon and made it clear to her if my request did not work out, it was perfectly okay. The current situation took priority and I would deal with my breast issue at a later date. She reached in her pocket, pulled out her cell phone, and shot off a text. Within two minutes there was a return text. Little did I know that she shared an office with one of California's best breast cancer surgeons, and her experience was vast, as these can usually involve axillary node dissection. So how fortunate I am again. She graciously squeezed me into her schedule once my visit with my oncology surgeon was complete. This is one of those moments that I view as a 'mountain being moved' for me. I may not have thought this before but today, in my current walk with HIM, this was Godsend. A blessing to me for sure. All good things come from above. I am convinced, once again, there are no coincidences.

> *"Have faith in God! If you have faith in God and don't doubt you can tell this mountain to get up and jump in the sea, and it will. Everything you ask in prayer will be yours, if you only have faith"*
> *Faith can move mountains.*
>
> JESUS SAYS THIS TO MARK 11:22-24

I walked on down to her office and was taken into an exam room. She did a complete physical examination. She could palpate the abscess within my right breast. She concluded it was wise to give it more time to reabsorb. Sometimes with surgery, there is the potential of introducing a new organism. But, since we already knew this abscess was a "sterile" abscess from previous cultures that had been taken, meaning there was no infection currently present, it was better to leave it alone at this time. But she had heard my story of how this all started and my concern for inflammatory breast cancer. So she went out of her way to get the tissue samples and 3D mammogram report sent to Stanford, and had them reviewed and retested by the pathologists there at Stanford. So I received a second opinion in the pathology department as well, that confirmed this was not cancer. I thanked her profusely for her diligence and expertise. I informed her my surgery was on the calendar for April 11th, she had mentioned if anything changed within my breast, my surgeon would give her a call. Again, that was impressive.

I would have my preop appointment with anesthesia the day before surgery and also the L-Dex test as mentioned, to get a baseline reading of cellular fluid. We would spend the night in town as we had done prior. I was ready to get this done. I requested they call me if they had a cancellation any sooner. Once my mind is made up about something, people say I am relentless. It is what I call 'missile lock.'

They ordered my first set for both the PET scan and brain MRI that needed to be done before the surgery. I knew it would be difficult for me to get these tests done some time after the surgery. Plus, I really wanted to go into surgery knowing these two tests were already negative. There was anxious moments in the results of these tests, as none of us were expecting my SLN biopsy to be positive. But I did have a pit in my stomach on that one. I seem to be defying the odds, and it was unsettling. I did not, however, have a pit in my gut for these two tests. I had been feeling perfectly normal up until now. Both tests were completed by mid to late March. We as a family had continued in prayer. Family and friends had been kept in the loop, as I really wanted as many thoughts and prayers as I could get. We were praying for all tests results to be negative for the potential spread of melanoma. Still awaiting on news of results on March 31st, I had written a prayer to my family and texted it to them.

Prayer to My Family ~ I pray for the glorious riches God our Father has offered us, with no strings attached, but for us to accept His Gift of unending Love and receive His Peace - which transcends all understanding, knowing that through the ransom paid for the forgiveness of all sin by His Son, Jesus Christ, and with the Power of the Holy Spirit filling each of you to your innermost being. May these Glorious Gifts in all their abundance spill over to your children and be recognized in you and by all who know you. Mom

My husband responded via text:

"You will keep in Perfect Peace those whose minds are steadfast because they trust in You. Trust in the Lord, forever, for the Lord, the Lord Himself, is the Rock eternal,"

ISAIAH 26:3–4

My daughter responded:

"I will give you peace. I will not give you what the world gives you. Do not let your hearts be troubled, Do not be afraid,"

JOHN 14:27

Spiritual Pearl ~ Four

In the week awaiting those test results, the peace I found in reading the scripture daily and reading my devotional kept me focused on my new journey of faith. I needed to trust and catch the updrafts of His grace on my new wings of faith. If I am going to obsess about something, why wouldn't I want to obsess about the greatest thing in the world! I remember hearing this once. He has promised to be with me. I can't say what changed, but I looked forward to spending time with any of my chosen resources. It gave me strength and courage every day. There was so much rich scripture I was discovering for the first time. Maybe I had read or heard it before, I don't know, but now with everything different in my life, it revealed its meaning. Every word was being spoken to me and I began to feel the joy deep within my heart. This joy was more intense than holding my firstborn in my arms or seeing my first grandchild for the first time. It was better than Christmas morning, and anyone who knows me knows I love everything about Christmas!

My day started with anticipation for what I would be taught from a teacher who doesn't need to learn anything and already knows all. I enjoyed what I felt was a relationship developing, like He was waiting for a visit. I would thank Him for all the blessings in my life, as I know everything I have that is good comes from Him. I was reading 'encouragement' every day. Things like:

> "*For everything God created is good, and nothing is to be rejected if it is received with thanksgiving.*"
>
> 1 Tim 4:4

HOW TO PRAY

Now I remember at some time in my Christian life, many years ago, a pastor explained how we should pray. It was an acronym that I could not recall. But my husband reminded me of it when we were discussing how I came to prayer. In my rawness of explaining it, I mentioned that first I **recognize** that He is my Almighty God, King above all Kings, Creator of Heaven and Earth. Then I **repent** and ask forgiveness of my sins, my grumblings and missed time away from Him. I follow this by **thanking** Him for all the good in my life and the blessings that are both apparent to me and not apparent, and many of the blessings yet to come. Lastly, I **submit my needs**. I sometimes don't even get to this part, as I can go on and on with thanking Him for so many things, not just in my life but in this world. That is my raw prayer model. But hey … check out the acronym; I actually did pretty well.

My husband explains the acronym ACTS in his way, but you can find versions for this online as well.

A = Adoration and acknowledge. Acknowledge that *"Praise be to God"* – Psalms 68–35. He is the most HIGH, Majestic, and King over all creation.

C = Confession. Confess your sins, transgressions, grumblings, and not making Him a priority. "*If we confess ours sins, He is faithful and just, and will forgive us our sins and purify us from all unrighteousness.*" – 1 John 1:9

T = Thanksgiving. Always *"Glorify Him with Thanksgiving."* – Psalms 69:30. Thank Him for His love, His faithfulness, His patience. Express gratitude for what He has done in your life and what He will do in your life. Thank Him for being your conscience, your counselor, and that inner voice. There are multitudes of blessings you enjoy.

S = Supplication. *"Present your requests to God"* – Philippians 4:6. Submit your requests to God no matter how small they seem to be. Do you really think any of your requests are too big for Him to handle? He holds the entire world in His hands.

This is an excellent way to start every morning with your cup of coffee and cell phones off. No distractions. Nothing is more annoying than when you are trying to have a meaningful conversation and you are interrupted by something. He deserves to have my undivided attention. I will be a model student and not interrupt His teachings. I know I will be blessed for this.

TEST RESULTS ARE IN

April 5th was a great day, and the day after my first swim and heavenly vision. My PET and MRI test results are in and I received news of my scans one week before my surgery. This was another very interesting day. I started my day with a daily devotional and in looking up the scripture Sarah Young got her inspiration from, it became another encouraging read on a day I really needed it. Once again, it seemed when one day brought more worry than another, scripture always provided the comfort I needed. Sometimes I need to just sit and practice the discipline of 'silence' while I am waiting, knowing He will understand me. I read:

> *"Yet the Lord longs to be gracious to you, He rises to show you compassion. For the Lord is a God of justice. Blessed are all who wait for Him!"*
> ISAIAH 30:15–18

I was trying to maintain a positive attitude after the PET scan and brain MRI until I heard the results. But these tests are so important to see if the cancer has travelled to other organs. No one was expecting my stage I to be in my lymph node, but my gut felt different. This would be additional diagnostic information for my physicians as well. So there is some anxiety that goes along with waiting for this kind of news. As we awaited the news, I pondered what my path would be. I felt we would be arriving at a fork in the road. If we went to the right, had good news, we could proceed with the surgery and try and get some normalcy back in our life. If we went to the left, bad news, we would have a bit more of a challenge ahead other than recovering from surgery's post-op course. I get reminded over and over this is completely out of my control. I have been gifted with capable organizational and multitasking abilities. But when you can't physically manipulate a circumstance, because you cannot touch it or control the outcome, this is very uncomfortable and tough to accept. There is no alternative other than I have to let go and allow what will be to be.

Holy Spirit Moment ~ Three

While surgery had been scheduled and this was a 'for sure' thing, the possibility of participating in the trial remained undecided. However, if I received this one particular medication in the trial, which is why I had been encouraged to consider the trial in the first place, I may rethink it. But as you recall when discussing immunotherapy, I did not have any hope in the outcome of taking these medications. My two friends had such a struggle with the risks associated with them. I said to my girls, "I have no 'hope stories' from people who have used these meds. Maybe if I had a hope story I would consider it more." The benefits just never seem to outweigh the risks for me, and I got nauseated every single time I thought about it. **The benefits may outweigh the risks for you, though. And the encouragement from your physician for individual therapy needs to be considered seriously, not what my choice is.**

April 5th was an interesting day because great things happened six days before my surgery. First, I received a 'hope story.' Out of the blue, I received a call from an FBI agent who was wanting to interview me as my name was given as a reference for a job from one of my friends' daughter. She desired to pursue a career with the agency post college graduation. He wanted to meet with me the following week at my home on Monday, April 10th. I apologized and said I could not meet with him, as I would be heading out of town and undergoing surgery. I asked if we could discuss any of this over the phone, as I knew this young woman and wanted to give her a good reference. He proceeded to ask me if I didn't mind sharing what kind of surgery I was having, that he would like to keep me in his prayers. Who does this over the phone, in a job reference conversation? He didn't even know me (well, he may have done a complete background check on me, I don't know. It is the FBI after all). He had a genuine tone in his voice, so I shared with him my upcoming surgery. He proceeded to tell me of one of his best buddies in the agency who had been diagnosed with malignant melanoma stage IV, and had metastasis to the lungs. See, again, there is always someone with a more difficult trek. His friend was treated with the trial drug, Keytruda, and is presently living a full cancer-free life. A 'hope story' with the Holy Spirit as the author spontaneously delivered to me?

He went on to tell me that he had his own health issues and believes in the power of prayer. He knew I was a nurse practitioner, because the common link was the candidate's mother and I had worked together in the past. He asked me several questions regarding this young woman and I answered them. I gave her a glowing recommendation. He wished me luck, said he would be praying for me and then said to me, "I am sure you have been a great influence to your patients, and I don't even know you." That was so kind. This was an out-of-the-blue phone call, and no coincidence again. The Holy Spirit paid another visit and provided me with a perfect stranger, a caring human being who believes and recognizes the power of prayer. He provided me with an out-of-the-blue 'hope story.' What are the chances of his story being about a friend with melanoma stage IV, given the medication I was considering? Some mathematical whiz can figure the odds of that happening out I'm sure. If I was going to consider any immunotherapy medication after the surgery, it would only be in the trial and only if I received the trial arm drug, Keytruda. By the way, upon her graduation, I learned she did get the job!

The second thing on April 5th that proved it to be a great day was the call from the oncologist. The call came in the early afternoon, right after my conversation with the FBI agent. Both my PET scan and brain MRI results were negative. They had been reviewed with me in detail. Thank you family and friends for all your prayers, and thank you Lord for answering them!

And of course the best thing came in the early morning as I sat and read the word, which provided me encouragement and hope before my day even started. How do we know that all that has transpired to date is not because of the prayer chain that started months ago? Was it the power of prayer that influenced my results? I don't know. And I don't know if the answer really matters to me. I know the test results could have swung the other direction as they do for some people, obviously. But I don't know if I would view it as a 'failure' in prayer. Because even if HE doesn't provide an outcome the way I hope it to be, my faith will still be in Him. In His plan for me is where I wish to be, as He is so worth my investment. This is a very short time here on earth, and this great news cannot be taken for granted. I have a thankful heart for this day and what He provided in my 'three' gifts. I wonder what He is still wanting to do with me.

My journey towards heaven is my daily walk.

CHAPTER TWELVE

PREPARING FOR SURGERY AND FINDING PEACE

THE WEEK OF SURGERY, April 5 – April 10

Take nothing for granted. I continued daily with readings from here and there and also listened to more online sermons, taking notes and journaling. Still no book idea had even been a thought. As the surgery date was getting closer, the words I had been absorbed in became more and more profound. I was consumed. Day after day my maturing faith has allowed peace to make its presence known. My heart was calming as my trust was building. These were my notes in my journal the week before. Love so amazing. And all the while, behind the scenes, He was quieting my heart and my mind, preparing me for surgery. My awesome Chief of Staff.

April 7th, "*He who receive Him, to all who believed in His name, He gave the right to become children of God. Born to God. Do not let yourself reject Him. For you will have One Hope.*"

CHRISTIAN RADIO

There is some unsettling of nerves with any impending surgery. It is human and it's okay. I am doing pretty well on this day.

April 8th, "*In one single moment, never to be repeated, was atonement for everyone. The just and the unjust. God is ready to receive us, at any time He will welcome us. It is up to us to receive Him by faith and follow His Word. Jesus Christ sitting at the right hand of the Father waiting for us, and He knows exactly when we are going to arrive. Right on time!*"

PASTOR CHARLES STANLEY

These few days leading up to my 'big surgery' were so inspirational and reassuring to me as I continued to learn and focus on His Word. I was confident I would not be left alone. While I was waiting in the preop room, I could think about all the wonderful scripture that I have read. He promises that nothing, absolutely nothing, can separate us from the love of God that is in Jesus. He promises to watch over us wherever we go and will not leave us, until His promise has been fulfilled for each of us. He will stick around so that His plan for each one of us may unfold independent and uniquely from each other. It will be for His purpose if we remain focused on Him and allow Him to work through us. He has never changed throughout all the ages, and forever more He will never change. He has never readjusted His plan. The adjustment comes from within us as we make room for Him to work, so the Will of God may be completed.

"*For I am convinced that neither death nor life, neither angels nor demons, neither present nor future, nor any powers, neither height nor depth, nor anything else in all creation, will be able to separate us from the love of God that is in Christ Jesus our Lord,*"

ROMANS: 38:39

"*I am with you and will watch over you wherever you go and I will bring you back to the land. I will not leave you until I have done what I have promised you.*"

GENESIS 28:15

"Jesus Christ is the same yesterday, and today and forever,"

HEBREWS 13:8

"And we know that in all good things God works for the good of those who love him, who have been called according to His purpose,"

ROMANS 8:28

"If God is with us, who can be against,"

ROMANS 8:31

This was my meditation, my yoga for the mind. What exquisite literary truths. All this nourishment before a surgery, when I had yet to know how my life would change once it was said and done. It didn't weigh as heavy for me, as my quiet confidence lay with His provision and guidance for me through this journey. There isn't anything that can separate or beat out of me, my love for this Omnipotent God. Whatever awaited me, He had suffered so much more. Then I randomly opened my women's devotional. Again I read a favorite:

"Be still and know that I am God,"

PSALM 46:10

WHAT IS TRUST

Trust is only experienced when your 'faith meter' reaches 100 percent, and there is not a moment of hesitation or doubt in your mind or heart about the existence of an Omnipotent God. It is an independently accepted 'gift of surrender to God,' recognizing His plan for you is greater than you can possibly understand. This trust as defined by me.

So when circumstances seem so huge and I feel caught between what I want and what He offers, I choose Him to lead me in the direction of His choosing. He is able! This is His world, He made it, and He controls it. Having sacrificed His very life for me, I should 'trust' in Him with every detail of mine. He may not show us what lies ahead, but He will equip us for the journey. I am going into this surgery with a different frame of mind from that with my SLN biopsy surgery. I really was at peace the day before surgery. No matter what the outcome. *Because now*, I thought, *I may have more of an understanding into 'why' His Will needs to supersede mine. It would be a reason for His glory and His glory alone. Do with me as you wish. I Trust You.*

Where is this coming from? How do I trust something with all of my heart? When I read or hear something devastating in the news, I usually will turn to the station or news team that I feel will bring me the truth to confirm it. I do not believe everything I hear, but sometimes I will put extra effort and energy into finding out the truth. Sometimes the effort is just enough to satisfy my curiosity. What about you? Do you need to then see it with your own eyes, or is reading about it enough? There are many things we will never see but we know must exist, because we have heard of them or have seen pictures. Taking the steps in faith for me was a time of discovery. Once the discovery was made, there was a spark that slowly ignited and I could feel it within my soul. As I trusted Him more, I could gradually let go of the controls I thought I had. I realized in order to trust in something or someone, I must first invest some quality time in learning more about it, and then I need to respect it. Just as I would anything else. The same principle applies here. Now imagine if you explored what faith could mean to you, and that 'WHO' you wanted to learn more about would never disappoint you. Never ever. Baby steps to start—that is what I did. First the investing and respecting my walk of faith, then peace and trust slowly emerged and a flame began to burn within me.

This feeling of the overwhelming love He has for me is the direct result of what I guess I have been fueling. He has the flame started, but every flame burns down and goes out. To keep it burning, it needs attention. Like I have mentioned, I have been a believer ever since I can remember, but the time I have spent getting to know Him is but a glimpse into what He is ALL about. I have been nurturing this relationship daily, for this has been my daily bread. This bread has fueled the fire, my courage, strength, and my love. It has to be nurtured daily. And by inviting Him in, I realize I am not alone.

I just went from being a believer to being in a relationship with My Creator.

HEADING OVER FOR SURGERY DAY

We head over to Stanford early Monday morning before surgery, as I had a preop scheduled with anesthesia after lunch and needed to complete the L-Dex test. All the details of the preop were typical and went without a hitch. The L-Dex took about twenty seconds, literally. I was done for the day.

We had our eldest daughter, Lindsay, with us. She and her sister had worked out who would be their father's sidekick while I was in surgery. Many thanks to her amazing husband, Matthew, for tackling the 'mom and dad' role for two days while she was away. We got checked into the hotel and while my husband did some work in our room, my daughter and I rented a movie to watch in her room. We bought popcorn, fixed our pillows, and settled in to watch something. A comedy was our preference. We decided on *My Big Fat Greek Wedding 2*. It was funny and nice to laugh while passing the time. What a special day it was to have her all to ourselves. When I spoke to my two-and-a-half-year-old grandson, Hawkeye, on the phone that evening at dinner I said, "I really appreciate you letting Mommy come and be with me." He said after a slight pause, "Well, you're welcome, Gigi." The blessings keep pouring in. Being a grandparent is just the best thing ever.

I had asked my younger daughter, Kendyl, to be in prayer for me as well. She said without question she would. She ended up being in prayer for me off and on all day long. She was being kept in the loop by frequent texts from either my husband or her sister. I did miss her not being there, but knowing she was praying for me was really all I needed. I knew my little family would be praying for me. The day before surgery, I spent time writing down some of my favorite spiritual truths. I decided to complete a prayer for myself using a compilation of truths that I learned and loved reading about. But more importantly I trusted in their promise. So I read this prayer the evening before my surgery and the morning of it for the three of us. I had it printed out and took it with me so I could focus on these promises anytime. These are my favorite spiritual truths and it reads:

Favorite Spiritual Truths Prayer

Oh Father, How great Thou are!
Forgive me of my sins, iniquities, grumblings, and times away
from You.
You already know how this day and circumstance unfolds,
and I trust and give thanks for what You are going to do.
I know You have the best for those who wait for You and are
obedient.
Father, You are my Refuge, Strength, my Companion and
Provider.
I will not fear, for You will never leave me and will be holding my
right hand.
I will be still and let Your peace guard my heart and mind,
because You are God.
You will give me the strength I need to meet the challenges of
the days ahead.
For Your test of my faith is to mold me for Your purpose and
Your plan is perfect!
I will be quiet in confidence as Your strength has its grip on me,
and I have felt the power of the Holy Spirit.
You are my "Known God,"
and I have hope in You through Jesus Christ my Savior!
I will walk with You always.
My Lord, My Savior, I will live by faith and trust in You all the
rest of my days.
Amen

SURGERY DAY- THE 'BIG' SURGERY

Well, today is the day. April 11, 2017. This will be one day in my book of life and I am trusting with an open heart for Him to do what He chooses. But it is also the day I have been dreading and the day I was looking forward to having behind me. *What will be in store for me this day?* I wonder. I had a very tranquil and untroubled feeling as I awoke. I had slept pretty well and felt rested. I read the prayer I had written one more time. This was going to be a same-day surgery, which I was so thankful for. Seriously, who enjoys being in the hospital? We parked and walked in holding hands, finding our way to the admission's office to get checked in. After the paper work was complete, we were all set to move on. The three of us waited until it was our turn to be called in for preop. The usual questions were asked, consents were signed. I changed into the usual hospital attire, now socks and a warm blanket, and I was set. The IV got started and running. The surgeon came in to say hello and I was sure to ask her if she got a good night sleep, had a good breakfast, and was ready to tackle this morning. She said she slept well and had eaten. She was ready to do this. She was just so precious.

My husband does not like discussing the 'what ifs,' as it is an uncomfortable physical experience for him, but it was really important to me to tell him how much I loved him and everything we have had together. I told my husband not to worry, as this was a win-win situation for me no matter what happened. I have always thought I would rather have a happy, short life span than a miserable longer one. The Lord put us together many years ago and must have known why. I was feeling calm and at that moment I placed ALL my trust in the Lord. The week prior to this surgery was a spiritual lead-up to this moment. A spiritual preop, so to speak. Was I so into prayer because I thought it would sway the outcome? I don't think so. I remember reading, "*It is impossible for you to have a need I cannot meet.*" So He will be here with me today. "*I can do all things through Him who gives me strength!*" And I can get through this, and the days, weeks, months and years ahead, whatever they may bring. Believe me when I say if He wasn't completely near and holding my right hand on this, I would have my heart pounding out of my chest, sweaty palms, feeling sick to my stomach, and be downright scared. I wasn't experiencing any of that. Like I had in the past. And this time, I did not get any medication until I was in the OR. So my peace was coming from within and confidently promoted by faith and trust.

This was going to be my third general anesthesia in five months and my blood pressure had been yo-yoing. Up, up, and way, way down. So I needed to have faith in the nursing staff to manage this throughout. I have been in the recovery room before in past surgeries, and though not quite awake from anesthesia, I could hear every word the nurses were saying. Once I heard, "Her blood pressure is really low at 74/48, do you think we should call the doctor?" I am saying in my head, *Well, would you at least open my IV full blast while you decide! That may help!* When I awoke, I mentioned that I had heard them. They were so surprised. So this third time under general anesthesia in five months and how I would tolerate it had been on my mind. Again, *Trust in the God you know is near*, I told myself. This is a win-win.

The time had come when they asked my husband and daughter to leave the room. I received my 'see you later' kisses and they exited the room, behind the curtain. They were gone. They would go wait in the family post-surgery waiting room. There were televisions and a marquee-like board that had many different numbers on it, correlating to a given patient. I had a number, and my family could follow this number as it moved from preop, into the surgery room, and then on to the recovery room. They could see the progression as I was transferred through these areas.

Spiritual Pearl ~ Five

So here I was, waiting. I was lying on the gurney alone, the curtains drawn all around me. My IV running, I was warm and calm. Silence. I began with my prayer. Everyone should memorize this one scripture—it saved me.

"The Lord is near, do not be anxious about anything, but in every situation, by prayer and petition, and with thanksgiving, present your requests to God, whose peace transcends all understanding, and will guard you hearts and minds, through Christ Jesus,"

PHIL 4:5–7

Then I did something I wasn't expecting. While lying there alone, I said aloud, "You say you have me by my right hand; well, I say to You—hold me now by my right hand." I lifted my right hand and turned it palm facing up. I continued, "Here is my right hand." I looked down at my hand: I felt nothing. I left it palm facing up until I can't remember. But I was really calm. Then I scooted over to the left side of my gurney as far as I could, to make room. I said, "Jesus, I am asking you to sit with me on my gurney (and I patted the right side of the bed that I had opened up for Him). Be here in the OR with me."

It seemed like I was by myself for a long time. I was lying quiet, still and alone, or was I? Then an operating room nurse came in and said it was time. She asked if I was ready to go. Then I did something else I have never done before: I said, "I am ready to go, but there will be an extra person in the OR with us today." She said, "Really, who?" I said, "Jesus Christ is sitting right here beside me right now." She must have thought I was crazy or unstable, but I didn't care for one minute what she thought. In that very moment, my mind had never been clearer. My declaration: Christ was with me and peace surrounded me. She looked at me and said, "I am okay with that."

So she wheeled me into the operating room, where I could see all kinds of people scurrying about for last-minute preparations. I was instructed to scoot over to the operating table, so I did. I tried to scoot far enough over to make room for my Jesus, but that bed was narrower than the gurney I was on. Once I was on the operating room table, I remember purposefully sitting straight up, looking all over the room to see if I could see anything that may seem spiritual—I guess. I was on heightened awareness and I thought He may be waiting somewhere within the room. But I couldn't see anything unusual. I was just really calm. The anesthesiologist said, "Lita, it is time to lie back now." So I laid my head gently down. He didn't even ask me to count. That is all I remember. In all the past surgeries I have ever had, I never once sat straight up on the gurney.

When we are attentive to Him in the manner He deserves, we receive the glorious gift of His Perfect Peace. The hours must have dragged on for my 'three musketeers' awaiting any news. That is what we would call ourselves when one of us needed something: the remaining three were the musketeers. We all knew what the three musketeers meant: 'We are go!'

As I groggily and slowly awoke in recovery, the first thing I did was raise my arm. I raised it as high up as I could. The nurses made me put it back down. Thank you, God, my Chief of Staff! I can move my arm, which means the nerves have been protected. Just as my surgeon had promised. It would be her job to protect them, and she did just that. I could swim. One day. Several more hours went by, as it took time for me to come out of the anesthesia. But soon I was changing back into my casual clothes. Good ole yoga pants. I noticed the suction bulb was draining. The other end of the bulb tubing was lying directly in the midst of where she had just completed surgery, and was stitched in place for stability. The suction bulb has a job to do: drain the buildup of lymph fluid, which would collect and require drainage over the next week or two. We clipped it to my shirt; this would become my new friend for a couple of weeks. The nurse reviewed all the post-op instructions on how to empty and log the drainage within the bulb and care for the incision site. My husband was paying close attention. *Cute,* I thought. The surgery had gone well, without complications, and I did not hear any conversation from the recovery nurses while I was not yet awake. I couldn't wait to get home. I couldn't wait to hear my younger daughter's voice either.

We arrived home safely. My family and friends were all notified of the successful surgery thus far. The outpouring of love and concern was heart-felt and overwhelming. I was grateful not only to love so many people, but to have felt the love back from them during this challenging time in my life. I got settled into my bed, and mentioned to my husband I wanted to speak to Kendyl. She was on the phone before I knew it. With a raspy voice I said, "Good to hear your voice. Did you pray for me today?" She said she was in prayer off and on all the while I was in surgery and after. She mentioned that either her sister or her father were keeping her informed throughout the day, through texts or a quick conversation. We had some small talk and I filled her in on how I was feeling. Groggy and sore.

IDENTICAL VISIONS

Now Kendyl has had visions on occasion, as I have in the past. Lindsay does have very vivid dreams, but I don't think she experiences visions. There was one occasion I can recall where all three of us spoke of the exact same dream. Again, it was received in the heart of the night. True story. We all had a vision where their grandfather, my father-in-law, was sitting on a bench at our local mall. We were entering the mall when we saw him smiling back at us. As if wanting to say hello. He was wearing clothing we had seen him in many times before—a light shirt with his beige sweater vest, khaki brown pants, and brown shoes. He was healthy in appearance and had a grand smile on his face. He had a great smile when he was really happy. And then that was it. There were no hugs or even dialogue, just a very warm, pleasant smile and silent greeting full of love. He looked very much like he did when I first met him at fifteen years of age.

This first vision or dream for all of us, however you want to think of it, came one year or so after he succumbed to cancer. He battled, and I mean battled, difficulties for the last three of his ten-year fight. This is the type of cancer and battle I know bring the difficulties with them. I do not compare my trek with those who fight like he did. I was fortunate with mine being caught early. It was 2010 that he passed and in this same year, we all had the same vision of him sitting on the bench at the mall, smiling as we walked in. I had experienced another vision of him later in that year, in a dream I suppose, but I was walking into my home and there he was sitting on my couch, reading, with that grand smile on his face. I said, "I have missed you so much. Good to see you." There was no dialogue on his part, just a warm, pleasant smile once again. That was all there was to it.

CHAPTER THIRTEEN

GRAND ORCHESTRATION

MY DAUGHTER'S PRAYER TIME REVEAL

As Kendyl and I started talking, I told her I was doing fine. I was sore, but not in much discomfort—as yet. That was all I shared with her. With much energy in her voice, she began telling me how she prayed and was in deep prayer without distractions. She went on to explain that she had had a vision. She was glad to hear my voice and excited to share with me, so I listened. Then I listened more intently as she shared with me without hesitation that she was one hundred percent confident I was going to be all right. She said she just knew, because it had been revealed by the Holy Spirit who surrounded her with the vision. This is her testimony.

Kendyl's Testimony and Holy Spirit Moment ~ Four

To say this past year has brought the greatest spiritual test of my life would be an understatement. When I received the news my mother had stage III A melanoma after her SLN biopsy, it rang through me like a shock wave. For the first time in my life, I was brought to my knees. In disbelief but in prayer, with the Lord I've served since I was nine years old right there with me. His presence I felt, reminiscent of the time I had emergency C-section with my first daughter. My life and my unborn baby's life were hanging in the balance. I was afraid, but I had been in prayer with my Jesus and felt He was near. My Savior, my mother, and one fantastic nurse are the reasons why both my daughter and I are fine. I felt His presence through the chaos then, just like I did when I got the "news" and was brought to my knees. I feel His presence in my prayers.

After the positive news for her SLN biopsy and as I was on my knees, I wept uncontrollably for this beautiful woman I hold so dear to my heart. I was not sad for myself, but was experiencing deeper sorrow for her and my father as they would have to tackle this. The world has shown us how horrible cancer can be. Our entire family witnessed its death grip with the loss of my beloved grandfather, Bapa, who passed in 2010. My greatest wish while on this earth is not for money, cars, or big fancy houses, but for no other family member to have to suffer through the battle with a deadly cancer. I knew how serious melanoma could be: we had family discussions about it, as my mother made sure my sister and I saw our dermatologist right after her initial diagnosis. And here I was on my knees, facing my biggest fear head on. As I prayed and cried out to Him, I heard my Lord say, "Be calm, I am here. She will be well." In that moment my cries subsided, my breathing slowed, and a wave of peace came across my body. The road to wellness undefined for what may await her. But now I needed to make a decision: do I dwell on what is out of my control, or do I choose to believe what He just promised me? I did hear Him speak, and He said, "She will be well." I never shared this first vision with anyone, because as time went on, I wasn't sure if I was wishing it or it was real.

Prior to this morning of her 'big' surgery, she asked me to be in prayer again. While in prayer, as I could not be with her but in spirit, I would never forget this day. It was a day I would cherish the rest of my life, as the Holy Spirit shone brighter and was more brilliant than ever before. I began in prayer when I knew she would be in preop. I prayed the Lord would grant her peace and calm her soul. I could see her lying on the gurney in the preop room, and sitting on the edge of the gurney next to her was Jesus Christ. He was facing her and gently touching her legs. I guess as a sign of affection and control. He was holding her, He had this. He was sitting as if ready to take a ride into the operating room. Amidst all my worries: would they get all the cancer? Would there be more cancer somewhere else? Would she lose the use of her arm, mighty swimmer that she is? Would she be able to hold her grandbabies again? Would she lose her personality? And on and on the worries went. But when I saw Jesus sitting with her in the brightest light, my worries vanished immediately. As the hours passed, I continued in my prayers. I knew she was in surgery now, and my prayer went from peace and comfort to praying for complete healing and wellness for her.

That was when the second and most powerful vision came. During this time, the Holy Spirit blessed me with another incredible vision. There my mother was in the operating room undergoing surgery, with Jesus still sitting at the edge of the gurney, and I noticed my grandfather, Bapa, was pacing around the room. He was slowly walking around the operating room, his hands behind his back and taking quick glances at all the monitors. Suddenly Jesus got up, walked around to her left arm, and placed His hand right through her shoulder as if removing the bad that was there and healing her. I knew at that moment in prayer that not only would she be able to use her arm, but she would not have any more traces of cancer.

I did not share either of these visions with my husband, father, or sister as I wasn't sure if I imagined it all "in my head," which scared me. Or was this all real, again? What if I am wrong? So I dared not speak of this until I know she was out of surgery. But as I thought about it all, I believe in my Lord and all He brought me that day, so I knew it had to be true. I got the call saying mom was doing great, just as He Promised me it would be. I still didn't say anything until I spoke to my mother that night before she went to bed. The week that followed she had pain, but when the news of no more cancer being in the lymph nodes came, His Promise rang true again.

I suppose we worry more when we love someone so deeply. I really did try to hold onto the promise of "She will be well." Every time my mother had a brain MRI or a PET scan, that darn worry crept in. This last PET scan for some reason was worrying me. It was an early Sunday morning in December when I had a nightmare about her having cancer again. Lying there with my eyes tightly shut and terrified of the nightmare I just had, I began to pray to my sweet Jesus. As I prayed, a bright light came into my vision. As my eyes were closed, it passed me on the left side. I said, "Is that you, Holy Spirit?" He then spoke to me and said, "My child, what have I told you? She is well." I immediately asked for forgiveness for doubting Him, and my prayers turned to praise. I knew in that moment her PET scan would be negative. The next day, I got the news from my mother that it was in fact negative.

The spiritual journey this past year has taken us on has been a gift. Fancy that: cancer a gift. The opportunity to experience our Lord's Presence, hear His Words, and know His Peace is overwhelming. So while the year was a challenging one, it was also the most rewarding. As I have come to know my Savior better, He has drawn me in so close that I will never let go. The Lord blessed my relationship with my mother. Unconditional and pure love. He chose her to be my mother and at times I felt I could feel her pain. I watched her get up out of bed every day and still live her life with this burden of staying ahead of this and the daily discomfort with her arm. I admire her strength even if she doesn't think she is being strong. She has chosen faith, hope, and love instead of doom and despair. I look forward to the day where I can say, "Why me, Lord? Why was I the one who so richly experienced Your Presence and got to be the one to reveal and share in the good news and hope You would have for her?"

I asked my daughter Kendyl to put into her own words how she remembered both of these experiences in prayer unfolding. With only minimal editing, those were her words. And this was yet another Holy-Spirit moment for this family. When I listened to her share with me her time in prayer and the power it revealed, I was in awe. I felt so touched by Jesus at that moment, and I mean physically touched. I immediately had chills all over my body, and my eyes welled up with tears. I realized while I did not 'feel' the sensation of Him actually touching my hand when I asked Him to, He had taken a seat next to me. No wonder I had no fear at all. He is here and He keeps His promise to us. Once she had finished her prayer experience with me, as I had yet to share with her what I had asked of my Jesus in the preop room, I told her what I had done. Asking Jesus to sit with me before I went into surgery was the best thing I have ever done, as I trusted so completely and perfectly in that very moment—He was Glorified. This is unbelievable. I ask Him to sit with me and hold my right hand and He reveals this to her, and she sees it—while in prayer!

After we said our goodbyes on the phone, I called my husband into the bedroom and shared the conversation that Kendyl and I had just had. I shared with him everything I just shared with you, and I will continue to share it with everyone I can share it with. Reactions were interesting from person to person. But again I don't feel the need to be convincing, as this is my spiritual journey or revival. But it is made clear to me that we do all have a choice to make. If my experience can encourage even one person to try and seek Him out, I am confident they will find Him. I will elaborate more on the wonder of this moment later.

VISION LONG AGO - BUT A GLIMPSE

Which brings me to another vision, where only 'now' after this surgery I can see that my Lord may have given me a small glimpse into my future long ago. But He has His reasons for withholding how our future unfolds. This one occurred after my grandmother passed almost twenty-five years ago. Again, in the middle of the night. This dream was very clear and detailed: I was sitting upright on a gurney with a hospital gown on and I appeared to be older. Then suddenly there was a very bright figure approaching the right side of my gurney as I was sitting up. It was in the distance and moving towards me, like coming into view. As it closed in and became clearer, it was the face of Jesus. A white glow surrounded Him and flowed behind Him as He would pass me. He came straight toward me and gently passed me, brushing my right side, and He looked right into my eyes. Then He was gone. I remember sharing this with my husband and saying something to the effect, "I think I am going to be sick in the future requiring surgery." At that time I thought it might even be breast cancer. Now I have undergone many surgeries, probably more than half a dozen, and I have NEVER sat straight up on the gurney except for this last surgery. I have NEVER asked

Jesus to sit with me on my gurney except for this last surgery and on my right side, exactly where He passed me. It is what it IS.

I am sure there are people all over the world who have undoubtedly felt the presence of the Holy Spirit or Jesus Christ himself in a single profound and memorable moment. Maybe it was even their AH-HA moment. You don't forget these, and I am sure there are hundreds even more profound than mine. They will remain clear throughout the years to us. How can I ever forget something that has penetrated me to the very depth of my being? His presence can be felt here on earth as He gave us the Holy Spirit, and I for some reason experience visions off and on. Yes, I do believe in miracles.

But if you recall, my daughter's vision did not stop with just the sighting of Jesus on the gurney with me. I will expand more on it later. She noticed there was someone else in the operating room. He was walking around the room as if to make sure everyone was doing their job. It was her grandfather, my father-in-law. The same one we all saw in our dreams, known to all in this family as Bapa. Yes, our dear sweet Bapa, Robert or Bob, was in the operating room with me. Read on.

SPECIAL RELATIONSHIP

In order for this to make any sense to you, I must share a brief history surrounding my father-in-law, Bapa, and myself. We shared a very special connection. I revered him and he was like a father to me, as we had met when I was only fifteen. He was an anesthesiologist, and his opinion mattered very much to me. So when I wanted to attend nurse practitioner (NP) school, he really encouraged me to pursue this. I was concerned my being away at school would be too traumatic for my young girls. But he said I shouldn't worry, that the girls would be just fine and they were young, so this would be the time to do it. He volunteered that he and my mother-in-law would help out with the children while I was away. My husband was also supportive, and he was able to enjoy many home-cooked meals much as he did when he was a boy, which was a bonus! So off to NP school I went.

Bob had to struggle for about the last ten years of his life in his battle with cancer. The last three of those years were extremely difficult, and the last year was a nightmare. I had taken him to some of his appointments, which were at Stanford. We shared conversation and special moments that I will always cherish. One conversation I particularly remember. I asked him if he believed in God. And he said calmly, "I don't think so." I then asked him, "Then why did you take the entire family to church?" He replied, "Because isn't church a good thing?" He chose to introduce his entire family to church, the Bible, and most importantly, our Creator. Wow—right? What nonbeliever makes it a point to do this, just because they think church is a good thing? So with that mindset, I say just because we may doubt God's existence doesn't mean we shouldn't introduce our family to the possibility of His existence. Only then, wouldn't each of our children have at least heard the words 'Bible' and 'God'? Then they can make their own choice regarding walking on a journey by 'faith' towards Heaven or not.

But what is so amazing about the vision Kendyl had of her grandfather also in the operating room with me is the preorchestrated planning by my Lord to unveil clarity to this family. He had it years and years in the making—from the time I went to NP school, to the spiritual moment in the operating room. Actually it would have begun with six births, my in-laws, my parents, my husband, and my own. Sometimes we don't see or understand why something happens, and we may never understand and experience closure. Or it may be years later that a hint of reasoning as to the 'why' becomes clear. But our Lord orchestrated this moment to Perfection. Which is our Lord's way. Bob and I shared a history together, and I will forever be thankful for this bond. I had been encouraged by him to pursue my nurse practitioner license. Now almost thirty years later I am at Stanford. Diagnosed with cancer at Stanford, and having surgery for cancer at Stanford. I am confident he was in the room with me as well as Jesus Christ. I can just hear Jesus saying the morning of my surgery, "Hey, Bob, we are going on a field trip to your alma mater, so let's go." He loved walking the Stanford campus. Attended many football games where tailgating included having his kids with him. Taking them to these college games was his way of saying, "Someday, you will all go to college."

See, this grand orchestrated picture that was His original 'perfect' plan all along becomes even clearer yet.

While I had my own walk in this grand design, Bob had his. He was a bioscience major and graduated from Stanford in 1953. He was a graduate of Stanford medical school, class of '55. He was diagnosed at Stanford with cancer, had surgery and was treated at Stanford for cancer. He did not pass at Stanford, but at the Bruns Hospice house in Alamo, California, where I gladly volunteered and was honored to care for him the last seventy-two hours of his life. I loved him so much, and he would die in my arms. How rich is this—that he would be there for me, with Jesus, at Stanford, in the operating room? This was a place he had been before, and I with him. He had been in the operating rooms, having walked the back corridors for employees only many times before.

When I look at the entire picture, it starts to come together like a puzzle. Each piece is selected very carefully, to fit exactly. The pieces are specific to where they fit and are not interchangeable or the picture is skewed. Then slowly, as each piece is set in its proper place, the picture begins to emerge. This picture was made very clear to me.

The last piece of this puzzle for it 'to even become a vision' to my daughter and one that unveiled Bob's journey ending in Heaven was right before he passed. This last piece is truly important. If you have a single puzzle piece missing, that only comes to light when all the other pieces are accurately placed. The puzzle is disappointing, is not complete, and will never be complete unless that piece is found. If this last incident had not occurred, this puzzle or vision would not have occurred or taken on the profound significance it has.

Through the years Bob had read many books regarding Christianity, and had searched for the truth. He was mailed books by my husband on two different occasions. The first was called *Mere Christianity*—by C. S. Lewis, an Oxford professor—which he thought was an 'interesting read,' and the second book was called *The Language of God*. The latter of the two books was chosen when we reached out to our pastor and asked if he had a recommendation for a book that could be geared toward the scientific and highly intellectual mind? The *Language of God* was the recommendation (so I had read this for the first time, long ago, only to reread it this past year). So we mailed him a copy. It was within the last one or two years of his life that after he had read it, he e-mailed my husband thanking him for the book and wrote, 'It was a timely read.' We had a glimmer of hope that he may be starting to believe.

Bob would read many things, but we still could not tell if his doubt continued because we never saw him pray, and other than the conversation in the car I had with him, we never discussed it. I don't think he could conceptualize the act of 'faith.' He had a scientific mind, where the proof and facts were revealed within theorems and equations. There were so many questions he would love to ask Our Lord. He needed answers for all the 'whys' that he just didn't understand. Like why do children get cancer? Or why does God, who is good, let bad things happen to good people? Just a couple we all remember him asking. Legitimate questions: I don't have an answer for either. Almost as if these 'why questions,' this bad stuff, was proof that Jesus simply did not exist.

The missing piece that is at last found to complete this puzzle occurred in the last twelve hours of his life. I had been with him day and night for seventy-two hours. But the last twelve hours, I witnessed him raise his 'right hand' *three* times to the heavens. As if to be shaking hands, which was how he typically greeted you. But I always wondered who he was shaking hands with. Or maybe, who was welcoming him? Why three times in twelve hours? Now, numbers have a significance in the Bible, and so does the number *three*. The significance of the number *three* can be found in any NIV Bible, and it signifies several things. These are but a few and first is the obvious, the Trinity of Persons in the Godhead: God the Father, Jesus Christ, His one and only Son, and the Holy Spirit. The *three* Wise men, Jesus Christ himself saying in Luke 22:34, "*I tell you Peter, the rooster will not crow this day, until you have denied three times that you know Me.*" Also, there were *three* crosses on Calvary's hill at the crucifixion. Jesus is thought to have passed at *three* o'clock, and then *three* hours of darkness fell on the world after His soul left Him. The number three is also associated with the resurrection, where God raised Christ up on the *third* day. So, to me, raising his right hand to the

Heavens three times before He passed is symbolic. This is the last piece to the puzzle found. But it has not been placed within the puzzle as yet.

In the days before his death, his family would come and visit him at the hospice house. His youngest daughter, Kim, had been a believer since her early teen years. She was a disciple of Jesus, as she never ever hesitated sharing the good news, the Word, with anyone and everyone. He would ask me if Kim was coming back, I told him she would be back in the afternoon. Every single time she walked through the door, I watched his face light up. He would smile so wide and was so glad to see her. She was his baby girl, but I could tell something inside him sparked, unlike his reaction with any of his other kids. He most definitely loved them all, but she had something that would follow her through the door. She brought the Holy Spirit in with her. It was almost as if she had a spiritual aura around her. She had a halo glow over her head and, as she approached him, his eyes would follow her around the room. She had prayed with him, read scripture (he declined offers for readings from anyone else), and she had asked him at one point if he believed in Jesus Christ as his Savior. She states he had given a nod indicating yes. But in talking to her after his death two years later, she seemed hesitant and unsure if she really witnessed this action. When she shared this uncertainty with me and my husband, I informed her of what I had witnessed every time she entered the room at the hospice house, as I mentioned to you. She was an angel visiting him every time she came, and he knew it. I am convinced. The Holy Spirit had surrounded her, and God loved her obedience to Him and His Word. We all had glimmers of hope, but we were all unsure if he really had accepted Christ.

With the remainder of the family gone, my husband in the waiting room at the hospice house as this was extremely difficult for him to witness, I was the only one by his bedside. In the minutes before he passed, one of the nurses asked him if he wanted to see Jesus. And with his eyes open looking at her, he very slowly nodded his head. I witnessed this. While he was in the last moment of his journey here on earth, and before his last breath, I am pretty sure he had accepted Jesus Christ. With tears starting to stream down my face, I wrapped my arms around his head and holding one hand, I said, "Lord, please have mercy on this man who introduced his entire family to

You. He searched for You almost all his life and maybe still has doubts with your existence." Then I recited the Lord's Prayer. And I cried harder.

My hope is the mercy our Lord has. He has promised even in our very last breathe that He will receive us, lovingly. The last puzzle piece has now been placed to complete this beautiful life's puzzle that has interfaced and richly blessed my personal journey here on earth. I will not ignore or forget that it was Jesus Christ who had made all these special moments happen. For He brought Bob into my life from the beginning, as I fell in love with his son, Scott. And it was Jesus who chose Bob to escort Him on this amazing field trip to a Stanford operating room on April 11, 2017. All confirmed in one powerful vision.

SHARING MY JOURNAL ENTRY WITH FAMILY - EASTER

The uncertainty remained that he had accepted Christ with some of his grown children, but all were hopeful. I was certain. I shared with the family how most of the last seventy-two hours of his life went, including the last twelve hours and his nod, yes, all occurring seven years ago now. The Saturday of Easter weekend, which was only four days after my completed 'big surgery,' I had been journaling. My thoughts included this event and I felt compelled to share it. Easter is one of my favorite seasons of joyful praise, rebirth, and 'new life.' Christmas is my favorite season, for it is the birth of Salvation and Everlasting Hope. But this timing of His again, at Easter, I decided to share a portion of my journal with my brother and sisters in-law. So I took a picture of my journal and texted it to them what I had written. It is similar to what you have read here, but at the end I wrote, "What a reward and Gift our Jesus gave us all with this one vision that Kendyl had. In one moment and in one prayer by her, we see Bapa in the presence of Jesus. He must be in Heaven, otherwise this vision would never have been possible."

Within minutes of receiving my text and photo of my journal entry, I get a text from Kim. She stated she was with her husband and sitting in a meadow enjoying the new spring blossoms—and reading when she received my text. She said she started crying and tears of joy were streaming down her face as she read my entry aloud to her husband. She was so thankful I had shared something so personal. She said what a perfect Easter it will be. A few minutes after my exchange with Kim, I received a text from my sister-in-law, Stacey, who said she had just applied her mascara for the day and now it was running all down her face. But as she continued reading she did not care. She was overjoyed and thanked me for sharing my journal entry. The family needed this. It was a beautiful day, an unforgettable Easter full of His Mercy and Grace.

As I continued to write about my relationship with Bob and the care I gave for loving him as a father, it became even more profound to me. Sometimes the answer to prayer is years in the making for God and we don't even realize it. He has to orchestrate the placement of the right people, circumstance, and uses our trials for His Purpose. Then only with His Perfect timing—for it to become a flawless vision, dream, or answer to a prayer—can it unfold within His will. It was an answer to our prayer seven years after my father-in-law's death. Seven years. We all would choose to see this as being reassured that he walks with Jesus in Heaven. Something so beautiful, all that is good in my life, comes from God. This is my life story and I am blessed by all the spiritual moments I have been able to share in this book. Even at this stage in my cancer trek, I had not been led to write it down as a twofold topic in a book. I think my God knew it was coming, but I didn't know He would lead me to write. It is not my goal to convince anyone that this vision was real, for it was her vision and my life story with him, but only to share. I know it occurred, because 'it can' occur.

This is what I read the day of my 'big surgery.' The *same day* as Kendyl's vision while in prayer on April 11, which confirmed my day completely, and as if the Lord were confirming the entire experience and vision. It was simply worded:

There is an abundant Life in His Presence, today.

How would you explain this? Bob, my beloved father-in law, is the abundant Life in the presence of Jesus and the Almighty Father. That is how

I chose to interpret this, on this very significant day. No doubt about it. Another 'perfectly pertinent' read.

Holy Spirit Moment ~ Five

That night after my surgery as I slept, I felt someone touch my left lower leg at mid calf then gently caress it slowly down to my toes. As if to say, *There you go, I am going to go now. You are okay.* It woke me up and I looked at my husband thinking he must have needed something, but he was sound asleep and nowhere near me. I was sure it was the spirit of my father-in-law checking in on me and then I fell back asleep. I have not had a vision of him since. But I have really felt the impact of our extremely special time together here on earth. I am looking forward to seeing him again someday.

HURDLES WITHOUT PEACE

I mentioned the blessings with the vision providing hope this family needed, comforted by knowing my father-in-law was whole and with God. He did struggle and fought the good fight for ten years. He had been diagnosed with salivary cancer within months after his retirement. His treatments were grueling, with radiation therapy, throat-neck surgery, and he participated in a drug trial at Stanford, all for the benefit of science and to prolong his life. But believe me when I say we all witnessed this was a tough fight for him, especially the last one or two years, as my daughter also mentions. Cancer can be so ravishing. Many of you may have experienced this or witnessed this with a friend or loved ones already.

Everyone has a story; it is their 'dash.' Lived 1926–2010. The dash is everything in-between. This man was the last of the true gentlemen, a good man, and highly intelligent. A life well-lived. He loved and enjoyed his family, grandchildren, pets, work, and remained active with a variety of interests and outdoor activities. In the end phases of life, he had to cope with more issues than one can imagine. Every single area of his life was affected by this rot that cancer had on him. This is what I mean when I acknowledge my trek is not like those who suffer the full impact cancer can have on the 'entire' body. There are so many people who have a similar story. Watching cancer consume a person is a horrible sight to witness. I can't imagine having to endure it and fight like this.

He had become a vessel. Which, in the end, is what we do become. A vessel: a hollow container, or a means of transport from here to there. Cancer is so cruel. The treatments can be toxic, and enduring the daily limitations overwhelming. In the end, he had to let go of this world and move on to his final resting place. Heaven.

But when I compare my walk with faith, which helped guide me in tackling the challenges of my cancer and anyone's walk without faith, I can only wonder: how does anyone do it all alone? The excruciating hurdles and the daily pain are fatiguing in themselves. The daily grind: but with a God who gave me 'timely' strength, I was powerful. I had my moments feeling frustrated and discouraged, but the hopelessness one must feel with no light at the end of the tunnel I cannot fathom. It's utterly frightening to me. It makes me wonder if there is peace even for a moment when one has a devastating illness and no faith. Can one's mind not be stricken with worry, consumed with doubt, dark moments or thoughts? For this can happen even with faith in hand, as anybody can have an overwhelming day. Chronic conditions or not, surely physical and emotional symptoms present themselves as ongoing uphill battles, as well as the cancer battle itself.

The question was answered for me and peace was found when I embraced my 'faith' in a manner that is truly basic. All the baby steps I would take led to my amazing journey in this cancer trek. Can everyone experience this peace even in the most difficult of circumstance? If we let Him in, He Promises to be with us. Does meditation, yoga, hobbies, and other outlets provide enough sustenance on a daily basis? Where does the 'hope' lie?

I had experienced the envelopment of 'peace' as my trust in my new 'relationship' with Him was wholeheartedly appreciated just the day before my surgery, to be exact. But *confirmation* I was NEVER alone became real to me when my daughter shared in her vision in which she stated she saw Jesus sitting on the gurney with me. The nurses didn't see a 'physical presence' of

anyone else on the gurney. Nor did they witness 'someone else in the operating room with me' when I mentioned Jesus would be joining us in there,
as I was confident He was already sitting on the gurney with me. The reality
of asking Him to sit with me before my 'big' surgery on that amazing day is
when I felt the *Peace He brings with Him*. But her vision was proof He was
in fact there and I - was - not - alone.

I'm feeling led by the Holy Spirit and pulled to elaborate more in regards
to the vision and its message. When I scooted over to the left of my gurney,
to make room on my right side, I asked Him 'first' to sit with me, and I felt
the peace He brought with Him. But then He chose to bless Kendyl with
this vision while she was in prayer. A vision that fulfilled and validated my
request, all the while she was unaware of my request of Him in the first
place. And then He kept His Promise to be with me. Well, I had chills and
get chills every time I recall it. My eyes can still tear up. Aside from the
perfect peace that surrounded me before surgery, our conversation and this
testimony was the physical sensation experienced, instead of Him actually
touching my hand. When I asked Him to 'hold me by my right hand,' He
was ever present with me, and His Peace infused me. But instead of the
'sensation of the touch' of His hand to mine, His Will was to penetrate my
soul deeper yet, with unsurpassed peace and in a vision of Christ Jesus with
me—but through Kendyl's testimony. My Supreme Father was sitting with
little old me.

I remain in awe as I ponder over and over what this vision in its entirety
of promise means to me. Let yourself think about this for moment. Imagine
and picture yourself on a gurney, going through a major surgery, not knowing what the outcome will bring, or how your life might change, and you
find out Jesus was also sitting on your gurney, because someone showed you
a picture in which He in fact was there. Imagine how this must make you
feel. He knew me, and I am *just like you*. How amazing, love so amazing!
Here is a Polaroid of Jesus sitting with you—do you believe me now? If faith
was only that easy. Nope, now you need to decide for yourself in your own
time. This was the discovery confirmation—we are not alone! For me, this
was the day that confirmed I had gone from being a believer to being in a
relationship with my God. Being a believer, don't get me wrong, is where it

all begins, and they are both equally salvation-bound. But I am loving being a believer in a new relationship with my Almighty Friend.

I have wondered what if I would have felt the sensation of Him holding my right hand when I had asked Him to and the vision never occurred to Kendyl: would it have been more believable? Would you have believed it more? Would it have had the impact as opposed to the way it actually all unfolded? God knew exactly what He was doing and which avenue would hold the subtler but grandeur impact. He knew I would write this book long before I ever did, and what I would write about, for He provided me all the material and years of visions. But this vision and testimony full of promise, grace, and mercy—first for our beloved Bapa, coupled with seeing the face of Christ in the Heavens on that amazing first swim and the Holy Spirit moments—are the reasons, and powerful reasons, to engage in the writing of this book to begin with. How could I ever ignore sharing this amazing journey with you? For if there is even a remote possibility to ignite even a glimmer of curiosity and hope inside you, then my heart would not allow it, nor the Holy Spirit. For His Will, and a perfect one at that, is to be. The journey is always the story, part of my 'dash' now, both medical and spiritual, so it must be shared.

The second and third part of the vision cannot be ignored either. My father-in-law walking all around the operating room, looking at the monitors and making sure everyone was doing their jobs, is so him. He was great at his profession, anesthesiology. Patients loved him, the Sandman many would call him. He actually did the anesthesia for the miscarriage I had that I mentioned at the beginning of the book. I was sad, but it was a welcomed nap. I loved the fact the vision included him in the OR with me, as I had been with him on many occasions and even upon his death. I felt it a reward to be blessed with this part of the vision by Jesus. But most importantly it provided this family, by the grace of a Merciful God, a comfort knowing he was in fact in Heaven, with his bride at this time.

The third and also profound part of the vision is when she sees Jesus get up off the gurney and walk around to my left side and place His hand 'in' my left shoulder area as if to make sure all would be well. How can I not trust my arm to be well after this action? For my faith during this trek thus far has proven to be recognized and rewarded by Him, as I have learned to trust without question. So I believe with a little time for recovery, beyond the pain, drain, and tenderness of my scars, which should improve, already I can move it, lift it, and hopefully one day swim. She sees 'truth' and informs us the remaining lymph nodes must all be negative. Does my future medical well-being lie in this one action, in this one vision? Would His reaching in my axilla area have anything to do with the pathology report? In waiting, we will see if I am free of cancer at this time and perhaps forever more. If I trust without question, then the answer would be yes. I am well for as long as He wishes me to be well. I am well, but most importantly all is well with my soul!

Two portions of this vision were answers to prayer for my family: Bob's resting place and my spiritual and medical healing. But this powerful part of the vision may have an impact on all of you who are reading this, as it was meant for a broader audience. I think the vision of Him sitting on the gurney—providing the validity *we are not alone* even in our deepest despair—was the most important thing to share. There is much loneliness in this often cruel world. If loneliness isn't remedied, it can lead to mental restlessness. I've seen it. Oftentimes, loneliness suggests a state of being alone, solitude, or it may bring feelings of sadness and abandonment. Some loneliness, unfortunately, stem from being unloved. To have no one to 'love on' or feel 'loved from.' But loneliness, hopelessness, or feeling unworthy of being loved can be remedied. Just as I leaned on my God to visit with, He is waiting for you to do the same. He is with us in this world, but He is not of this world.

We never really know what is going on with a person standing right next to us or sitting in front of us. What type of struggles do they have on their plate, and how are they really coping? I honestly know there is peace that can be found in truly welcoming and understanding what faith means to you, as we are not alone in the world. And accepting and welcoming this Gift brings *love and forgiveness* also. Even as we sit by ourselves on our couch, or lie in our beds day after day, our struggle can be His burden. He wants us to release it all to Him. Knowing He is sitting next to us can be our comfort and love when we have no one else. Just knowing that the Glory of

God awaits us to the very end is a peace that is remedy itself. My struggle pales in comparison to so many others, maybe even to yours. For it is He who gives me strength and sustains my soul while I am only a vessel. I am convinced Bob is experiencing the Truth to that Promise now. Give me hurdles with peace instead, for I am not alone.

Spiritual Pearl ~ Six

Even right up until the end, we are a work in progress. Like an unfinished canvas. The Holy Spirit centered within us, helps us constantly evolve—if we allow it. Even as a vessel that cannot move, when every single thing is stripped away from us, if there is only a mustard seed of belief or love left for our Savior, we will experience our salvation in Heaven. There is no condemnation when we choose Him. We may not have lived a 'ransom worthy life,' for we all have sinned, but just the same, His only requirement is loving Him. He will take us—as we are. To be like a vine who nourishes its branches. We are the branches and as long as we abide on the vine, we are forever transformed and promised Eternal Life.

> *"I am the vine; you are the branches. If you remain in me and I in you, you will bear much fruit; apart from me you can do nothing. If you do not remain in me, you are like a branch that is thrown away and withers; such branches are picked up, thrown into the fire and burned. If you remain in me and my words remain in you, ask whatever you wish, and it will be done for you. This is to my Father's glory, that you bear much fruit, showing yourselves to be my disciples."*
>
> JOHN 15:5–8 NIV

So many promises fulfilled and unveiled as a reward for my simple, subtle act of trusting faith. I asked for Him to sit with me and He was there. Such a grand and powerful experience in my life, that only after sharing the story can you see where all the possibilities lie with Him, just as I have. To see His face in the heavens was another reward; I don't even know why He felt I was worthy of this, but I think now it was so I would include it here with you. The material—visions—He has provided for me is one of many stories out there I am sure. I am overwhelmed by this. So why not give God the miracle back and embrace the best thing that has ever impacted this world. I choose to remain on the vine.

CHAPTER FOURTEEN

THE FIRST FOUR WEEKS

POST-OP COMPLETE AXILLARY LYMPH NODE DISSECTION

First Day Post-Op

I had only taken half a tablet of Norco, which is a narcotic and used for pain, before I went to bed. I substituted Tylenol or Acetaminophen for my pain and took this regularly. I would rather be in pain than be nauseated, have my head spinning or be constipated for that matter. This would be a tough day and probably even the next couple of weeks or months. I was trying to keep my left arm elevated as much as I could throughout the day. This is really an important thing to do, as we need to fight gravity to help keep the swelling down. It's crucial to keep it elevated as much as possible in the beginning with this type of surgery. I was really diligent in following my post-op instructions. My bandages were secure under my arm, and the drain securely in place and doing its job. Bright red blood being drained. My throat was sore, I suspect again from the endotracheal tube needed for general anesthesia. I had good color in my arm and was clearly attuned to anything that would be a concern.

My pain was pretty severe. My arm would go through an array of mixed sensations. At times it felt like I had a tourniquet around my mid upper arm. The compression was excruciating, almost like I could shake and release the squeeze but no such luck. This would last for hours at a time. Then it would switch up and feel like a burning sensation, like my arm was on fire (not that I really know what that feels like), but this was an intense and deep heat sensation. It would be randomly followed by sensation of being as cold as ice, like it was a balloon ready to pop. I had severe tightness, achiness almost always in the upper arm. It also felt completely numb on the underside of the arm, and this area is still numb. Again an array of sensations, and I never could predict what was coming next. My side would ache by the rib cage, though it did not limit any deep breathing. I was tired and of course felt like I had just been run over by a Mack Truck. I protected my arm like you wouldn't believe; I did not want anyone to hit it or bump it. It would happen on occasion and I would go through the roof. I know this is nothing compared to what some people have to suffer through with their ailment, like my father-in-law had, but this is real pain, and I was thankful when I could fall asleep just to get some relief.

The sensations reminded me that I was very much alive. I think I took another half of a Norco the next night, and then that was it. I just gutted the pain out for months. I am still learning to tolerate it. Another adjustment. It is the most intense discomfort I have ever felt. At least with childbirth (and no meds), you knew the pain would be over once you delivered. So you can hang in there and you get a prize in the end! They told me it would be very different from the post-op course for the SLN surgery and they were right in regards to the pain! I can remember moaning off and on throughout the day and night. I was trying to control the pain with prayer and mind over matter. It was tough, as it just would not lighten up. I don't know why I am so stubborn when it comes to narcotics, but I am. I don't like how they mess with my head. But I would recommend to anyone else having this surgery: if you are more fearful of the pain and you would rather have the first couple of weeks be a blur, do it! Take your pain medication as prescribed. There is nothing wrong with that. Just remember, follow the dosing directions on the bottle, DO NOT OPERATE HEAVY MACHINERY and take a stool softener!

Now I had made arrangements for the next couple of days for someone to stay with me—you know, like a babysitter. In fact I asked my mother if she wouldn't mind babysitting me the day following surgery. She gladly helped me out and I can recall when she came over, she was wearing a beautiful blue floral print dress. With Easter approaching, I called her my "Little Blue Easter Egg." She had brought us dinner, and also brought me a gift. I unwrapped it and inside was a small porcelain white dove, symbolic of the Holy Spirit. I had shared my awareness of the Holy Spirit with her on several occasions, and I set the gift of my porcelain Holy Spirit in plain view, so I could look at it all day long. It is still there in plain view today as I write.

You can't do much for a long while with a bum arm (or wing) and a drainage bulb attached to your side. So to refocus, I would read my scripture notes or resources when I could. I have obviously spent much time in reading and studying His Promises, and with this one action there has been a reaction. In this active participation, I have been trying to build a 'better self.' There is a reaction in my heart and soul that overflows with joy as I get to know Him better. I have never done this before—give Him the attention He is deserving of. As I give him quality, uninterrupted time, I get excited as to what I might discover about Him today. Something is revealed daily as I sit and read that otherwise would not be known to me. I continue to be in awe with all that had transpired. I know my God is supposed to see me, He knows my physical pain and He knows what is ahead of me. I am confident He will provide all that is needed. It keeps me encouraged that He already knows how much I can tolerate. I didn't take but the one Norco for the entire recovery as I type this out ten months later. I don't say this to brag, I say this was unnecessary on my part when there is medication to aid with uncontrolled pain. Take it if you need it: really, it really, really does hurt!

I can meditate all day long on my newfound knowledge of my Friend. What will I discover today, I wonder? Today is a beautiful spring morning before Easter and I read: *God is the Only One who can satisfy the human heart*! I find this so far to ring true.

LOCAL ONCOLOGY VISIT AT ONE WEEK POST-OP

I am one week post-op, and my discomfort—pain—remains unchanged in my arm. I am exhausted. My appointment with my surgeon is scheduled for tomorrow, but only if my drainage has slowed. Today, however, I am heading to an appointment with my local oncologist. I still have my friend, the drain, or 'the ball' as my grandchildren would call it, in tow. It remains steady and draining a moderate amount of fluid, hence I doubt it will be pulled as yet. I continue to monitor the readings twice daily. The rule of thumb is the drain can be pulled or removed when the output is less than twenty milliliters in twenty-four hours for two days. Mine was continuing to output over one hundred and twenty milliliters daily. I was really hoping it would slow down, and just when I thought it showed signs of slowing, it picked up again. Otherwise, I was moving along a routine post-op course. No one goes through this type of surgery without pain. I expected to be in pain, as I really understood the physiology of it all. I think it would be safe to say there are varying degrees of normal for this type of surgery. No physician would be able to tell you exactly what you will experience post-operatively. But I can almost guarantee you will have pain. I am sure I will remind you of this many more times throughout this book.

For my appointment to my local oncologist, my daughter Lindsay will drive me. I am feeling shaky before my first outing. This was my first experience in taking a shower, and it has been an exhausting effort. My husband actually washed my hair the first time for me. It was so special feeling his loving, gentle touch. It was fun and he was precious. But he was back at work now and I would have to wash my own hair. I needed to be mindful of my suction bulb drain and tubing, so I hooked it to my necklace so it wouldn't freely hang down, swing, and get in my way, which was somewhat inhibiting. It does take two hands to wash my hair—I have medium-to-long thick hair. The simple task of washing my hair, my body, let alone shaving my legs, was proving to be fatiguing and lengthy. My arm is limited in its mobility, I cannot seem to hold it above my shoulders for but a few seconds and it becomes even tougher raising it over my head to shampoo my hair.

The pain is definitely there. That was the longest shower I have ever taken! I found I needed to lie down when I was done. With a towel on, I plopped on the bed. Well, not quite plopped, but every move I have to make is gingerly executed. I cannot even get dressed right after a shower: I am too exhausted to even try. It took over thirty-five to forty minutes just to get dressed, as I had to take frequent rests. *Oh, Lord, this has to get easier*, I would say to myself. *I can do this. I have to do this*. This is all a normal course for one week out. Remember, a total of twenty-five lymph nodes were removed. This will be felt—well, that's what I kept telling myself. And while the five-inch scar is on my upper back and another five-to-six-inch scar is under my arm pit area, it is the arm itself which proved to be more painful of the two, with significant Charley-horse-like cramping in the shoulder area every time I lifted it. Owie!

My daughter Lindsay picked me up to take me to my appointment, as I have not been cleared to drive. We walked in together, sat, and waited to be called, and I suddenly noticed I was the youngest one in the waiting room. There were times I would regress for a minute, because I could not believe this was real and I was sitting here. On the up note, I was looking forward to seeing Gloria again. Now Gloria was a former coworker of mine who I really enjoyed. I had not seen her in about ten years. When I initially called to make the appointment, I thought the voice on the other end sounded familiar but I couldn't place it. She did not let on that she knew it was me. So when I arrived for my very first visit, she greeted me with a big warm hug. Once again my wonderful Master placed a familiar face in front of me to comfort me.

Gloria greeted me again and we proceeded to the exam room. We went through the routine questions and answers. The doctor entered and after we chatted for a moment regarding how I was feeling, he examined me. After my examination, I informed him since my surgery was completed, I was qualified for this trial at Stanford. I mentioned they were encouraging me to partake in it and said I was the perfect candidate. I had told him about the trial drug, Keytruda, and the goal would be to try and get this drug in the trial arm. I asked if he thought there was any way he could be a satellite for this trial here in town, so I would not have to drive to Stanford weekly for this. He listened and took notes, but did not get my hopes up that he would be able to accomplish this. The deadline for me to start in the trial was the end of July. We would see what would transpire.

THE RESULTS—AGAIN

He had come in prepared and had read the surgical report. The pathology report that must have literally just been completed was available. I had not heard any news from my surgeon as yet, nor was I expecting him to have these results available, let alone reveal them to me. He said, "Well looks like all the remainder of the lymph nodes are negative for malignant melanoma, all twenty-two of them." Oh, my goodness! I hugged my daughter, who said, "Yay, Mom!" Did I just hear that all twenty-two nodes removed were negative for melanoma? What a blessing, and the confirmation was right there in the report. I wanted to see the report, so he showed me. It was printed right there in black and white. I made sure it was my name at the top of the report. Behold, it was true. Kendyl's vision revealed and Jesus's Promise was true—with just one swipe of His hand.

This surgery was not done in vain. But for additional diagnostics, more knowledge and now possibly may even prove to have been a therapeutic cure. Our prayers were answered. I think I have faith, but I clearly needed to see the results for myself. Humanistic response, medical person response to double-check the names. I don't know—that was what I always did, check the name twice and read the results once. He printed a copy for me. I continue to be a work in progress, I am unfinished, and I always will be. This is Him, the Potter, testing my faith and molding me like clay with His hand, aiming for perfection. Please continue Your work on me. He will never give up on me.

The news was reconfirmed the following morning by a call from my surgeon. What does this mean now? Does this change my prognosis? Do I still need to consider immunotherapy? All these questions warranted further discussion—next week. For now, I am thankful and rejoicing in His Promise. I will not think past today, no worries about tomorrow. There will be no distractions as He deserves my praise and prayers of Thanksgiving.

Every single time I had a circumstance that presented worry, my resources or scripture provided the answer for the day.

Today I read something to the effect, *All the world is filled with My Presence, be thankful for everything in your life. It is in your trials in this life that will bring Me even closer to you. You just have to whisper My name.*

Once again I needed to inform my entire team of support—family, friends and coworkers—with my good news. We must thank our awesome God. How truly blessed, profoundly blessed, I feel at this very moment. All my coworkers went out after work, had a drink, and cheered to the good news. This was so awesome. I felt touched.

THE WAY MAKER FOR THE TRIAL

Exactly six days after my visit with the local oncologist, I got a call from the oncology coordinator at Sutter Health with the cancer registry. Her name was Elise. She mentioned that my oncologist had reached out to her to see if she could get the trial guidelines moved here at Sutter Health Medical Center for a patient he had with malignant melanoma Cancer Stage III-A. She stated they did not currently have any patients with that diagnosis. But while she was in the process of making this happen, three new cases were revealed. The timing, she said, was weird that all of a sudden there were three more cases. She needed to make sure the lab could handle all the blood work and had the appropriate equipment. She obtained and reviewed the trial protocol and qualifying guidelines. She had the exact twenty-eight-page consent form I had been given at Stanford. She would be ready to review everything with me.

If you took the two days out for the weekend, it means she pulled this all together for me in less than seventy-two hours. I say "Wow" again. This is God making a way, for He is a 'Way Maker.' She scheduled my appointment that afternoon, and was prepared to review the twenty-eight-page consent form for the trial and was available to answer any questions I would have regarding the trial. I thanked her profusely for this preparation. I listened to her read the twenty-eight-page consent line by line and word for word.

She reviewed all the possible risks associated with the medications from the milder risks to the graver ones, and even death, just as I have reviewed before. I understood everything being of the medical mindset. This could be a life-changing decision, and not always for the better. As with any drug, it can attack perfectly healthy organs. As we sat discussing this, I had a tear stream down my cheek again. I began feeling stomach pangs and became nauseated. Another moment where I could not believe I was even sitting there with the local cancer registry coordinator. Oh, and this one tear thing, it just happens.

The appointment lasted about one-and-a-half hours. I asked many questions, but this one I remember: what if I change my mind? She was gracious and said just because she has the trial available does not mean I have to do it. But stated she was surprised that now she had several other patients with the same diagnosis, since she had pulled it all together. She had read my chart notes and knew what tests needed to be completed before I entered the trial. If all of the remainder testing returned within normal limits, I would qualify. God literally moved mountains for me through my oncologist and Elise. I could not believe it. See what I am saying? He is in everything. And since I am looking, I am really seeing His handiwork. Does He do this more often than we appreciate or recognize? He probably does. Now there may be other people who will have a trial available to them also, and maybe this was the reason for it all along.

That week, we had another family meeting to review the trial and all involved with it. In conclusion, the decision ended up being my own. I am waffling, but doubting I will participate. I will have an appointment with my Stanford oncologist at my four-week post-op visit to discuss this again. He will review with me my options now that it has been revealed the remainder of the nodes (my pearls) were all negative. I will wait for him to weigh in with his opinion. I was hoping he would have one.

TWO WEEKS POST-OP

It is almost two weeks now since my surgery. I continue to feel very tired, run-down, and seem to continue with my drainage output. My doctor cancelled my appointment as my drainage output was still too significant in volume that she would not pull the drain as yet. I would continue to manage my wound care and keep track of my suction drain output. But a new symptom is occurring: I am noticing that my left breast is showing signs of possible infection. The skin is red, the breast feels very heavy, and at times it appears yellow tint in color. I am sure it is full of lymphatic fluid, and almost twice the size of my other breast. I start on some antibiotics for now, and we watch and wait. My poor breasts.

I searched on the internet to see if anyone with the same type surgery has experienced this. I found only one and they weren't very detailed, and I couldn't tell how many lymph nodes they had excised either. It was at this time when I thought this writing needed to include some medical awareness, as I do believe there is a great variance of 'normal' post-op course. We know recovery will vary for each person. This makes perfect sense to be a possibility for occurrence. The lymph fluid is going to collect, and will flow to the area of least resistance, hence the soft tissue of the breast. The breast was becoming red because within the lymph fluid are impurities and protein, which may contribute to this. The circulation within the breast is different from the circulation anywhere else in the body. And from what I have read, there is a risk for mastitis in general with this type of surgery, so I have to stay aware. One more thing to pay attention to.

I would take pictures of my 'battle' wounds which were tender and drain insertion site at request of my doctor, as it was really important that there were no signs of infection, especially since the drain had to remain in place longer. I was getting discouraged as they had said it would be one to two weeks. I was at the two-week mark with no signs of the fluid collection slowing down. My armpit area was starting to feel fuller and more pronounced than before. Again, there can be such a huge variance for a 'normal' recovery. What happens to me, may not be what others experienced. But when you focus on the physiology of the circulatory system, in which the lymphatics are a part of it, the changes occurring do make sense. Not very comfortable, but is expected. I know the physicians cannot predict how our post-op course will be. But my nurse was right when she said this recovery will be a different and a long-term adjustment type of recovery, in comparison to the sentinel lymph node dissection surgery. My scars are tender. My breast is heavy, my body is changing. Two weeks out and I am getting a little discouraged, but no regrets.

As I continue my journaling, I have noted that my April 26th journal entry reads;

April 26[th·] for the past few days I have noted to be more teary than usual. I am not exactly sure why. For I certainly remain grateful for the good news of my remaining lymph nodes being negative. Perhaps it is because the possibility of a life-changing decision still looming over me with consideration of the trial or immunotherapy. Maybe because I've noticed that already two weeks out and my arm is more bothersome and for longer periods of time. The aching and burning seems to be more persistent. I am distracted by it, which is what I tried so hard last week not to do. Being distracted by my arm and side pain is not where I want to be, as it can continue all day long, nor do I want to focus on how my body looks. But it is my human behavior. Pain medication at this time is still Tylenol for me, as I guess I prefer to have discomfort instead of being sedated to control the pain. Again, taking pain-controlling medications is prescribed for a reason and it is not necessary to suffer. I don't know why I am so stubborn with this.

THE CANVAS

I stated earlier that another scar did not bother me. Well, that was then. Of course one would always choose a scar in trying to prevent an invasive melanoma, I know that. While I am recovering from my 'big' surgery, I am frustrated and feel overwhelmed with everything going on with my body, breast, and my tender large scars. I am sure the frustration comes from having to dress the wounds, and care for my suction ball drainage while experiencing significant fatigue, pain, and tenderness are all playing a role with these emotions, as it is a daily reminder of my current trek. It is all fatiguing.

But now as I write and think back, I recall moments where I hated my body. It felt as if it were failing me, in a way. I am hard on myself, as we women can often be. I have removed the burden of feeling like I needed to compete with maintaining a youthful appearance off my plate long ago. So with all my little 'jiggles,' my remaining freckles and these new scars, I wasn't liking what I was seeing in the mirror every day. It is a body disfigurement, in a way; it will never look the same. Not to the extreme that some people may experience, like the loss of a breast or limb, and I get that. Truly. But the scars and changes with our bodies is a reminder of our journey and the cancer we are trying to defeat, or have defeated.

When I finally felt like I could get out of the house, with my 'ball' in tow, I went shopping. I was not looking for anything in particular, just wanted to have a change of scenery. While I shopped, I came across a large, beautiful oil-on-canvas painting. It was a picture of the backside of a woman wearing a backless gown. Her hair was tousled up off her neck and her back was exposed and flawless. Her gown was full and flowed out behind her. I loved it. So I purchased it and would wait for my husband to hang it over our bed if he liked it. When my husband made it home from work, I asked him if he minded that a more feminine picture hang over our bed. I shared with him why I bought it. I told him when I saw her in the store, she reminded me we are all beautiful. I continued as I was holding back tears and my voice cracking, and said, "She reminded me that I am beautiful, and I would appreciate seeing her grace my wall every time I walked in our room." The sweet man that he is said, "Then I think she should stay if you feel beautiful, because you are beautiful." So he hung the picture over our bed. In all the forty-two years of being together, he never once has made me feel bad about myself or my appearance. He always said what he loved and found most attractive in me was my confidence.

Now as the days pass, she continues to be a daily visible reminder to me. I continued to spend time with my daily nourishment in my chosen resource and in doing so, very gradually over time, the frustration with my limitations in my arm, breast, and scars seemed to ease up. Fueling my mind with God's love changed my inner spirit. When I recalled those feelings of failure in my body I became so sad, but not because I was still dwelling on the difficulties. That overwhelming feeling was steadily being replaced with peace, love, and strength. The more time I spent in the word, the more they kept squeezing their way into my heart and mind. So while these emotions were easing up, I began to feel the sadness and guilt for having these thoughts to begin with. I know that sounds weird, and I remember sharing this with my mother. Of course she said I was being too hard on myself, as I was crying in her embrace. I probably was—of course I was! This too is a process to graduate through; it's an adjustment. I would recognize it was the maturing of my faith, as my focus was in Him alone. For how could I criticize His perfect design? God has made us in His image and He knows all of me. When we do not like ourselves, for whatever reason, He feels the pain. This must have touched and pained His heart, for He loves us just the way we are and knows who we will become. Just like the pearls are all unique, we are also. Fat, thin, strong, weak, young or old, scars or not … we are to love ourselves, just as He first loved us.

So two weeks out of a major surgery and with some time, I know I will be able to look past these scars as I process, welcome, and adjust to this change and accept a new normal for my body. While my freckles—that are just kisses from God as someone told me long ago—and these scars will forever be with me, I am grateful for the medical healing they provided me. These scars are my battle wounds, just as yours are also. He is equipping me for the challenge ahead and meets my daily needs because I am spending time with Him. As I persevere through each phase of recovery, it must include loving His change with my body in the weeks and months ahead of me. His Grace is appreciating all my baby steps in getting to know Him. I am confident it will defeat all my untoward emotions with the changes in my body, just as you may have already adjusted to yours.

When my manuscript was complete, I was committed to having it published. I realized I needed to start thinking about the cover for the book. I looked at covers of the many books I have lying around the house for ideas. Do I want florals, something abstract, spiritually simple, or just words on the cover? What do I want?

I walked back into my room, and there she was, already hanging over my bed. Suddenly this beautiful idea of recreating the canvas became my inspiration for the cover of this amazing journey I find myself on. But in considering the cover- I realized I had not included the sweet story that surrounded the purchase of the canvas to begin with. So I included it once the manuscript was complete.

For after almost thirty years in women's health and listening to all the negative feelings or misperceptions of oneself, women have. I concluded, we try too hard to please. Most misconceptions result from low self-esteem, for whatever reason or striving for perfection. We women are too hard on ourselves when it comes to appearances, weight, with hoping we can age gracefully to boot. Now place on top of that, having scars or disfigurements to accept as a welcomed change. So I wrote the story behind the painting and include it here. I am so glad I did.

As for the cover, it was the Holy Spirit paving the way once again. He puts an artist in my path. An acquaintance from church through the many years. One day Ragena reached out to me for a lunch date. We exchanged pleasantries, and got to know each other better in a short amount of time. I shared my journey, the book, and need for a cover artist. I could not believe she was an artist. She had some pictures of watercolors on her phone and shared them with me. They were beautiful! She encouraged me to attempt painting my vision for the cover. So she gave me a lesson, and then we shopped for paints, and the right paper for my attempt. I borrowed her brushes to complete the watercolor which graces the cover. I actually painted four versions of the cover.

So the final choice is my watercolor of 'My Girl'. She wears a more colorful gown, with her two reexcision scars on her back, a sleeve on her left arm, and a beautiful strand of pearls grace her neck. If you look close enough, you will see a dove in the upper right hand corner of the book. My precious new friend, and the Holy Spirit were my guides for the perfect cover.

Spiritual Pearl

So just as a mollusk creates a pure and rare gemstone while trying to protect itself from the irritant single grain of sand by coating it with calcium carbonate, I too must coat the irritant distractions and frustrations of my mind and scarred body by protecting and coating my heart with God's grace, a rarer gemstone yet. As I replenish my mind with the promises He has made to me, in the guarding of my heart, carrying my burdens, being my companion all while holding me by my right hand, do I recognize myself as a rare and valuable Child of God. My scars have turned to pearls, which will bring purity, wisdom, loyalty and will be graced forever by His Eternal love.

FOUR WEEKS POST-OP

God already knew the distractions of this world could make our minds spin. He understands the human mind is the most complex unit in our body, and it is also the most restless and unruly. The moment He gave us the freedom to choose, it became evident to Him we would have struggles with worry. He says, *Let Me control your mind, and focus on Me. Let My light permeate your thinking.* When the Holy Spirit is controlling our mind, we are filled with Life and Peace! When our mind is spinning, we cannot hear His voice. Simple thing to say, yet harder to do. These are His everlasting wishes for us each day as we journey through this life.

During the course of the next two weeks, I corresponded with my nurse and kept her updated on my recovery. The redness in my breast was stable but had continued to hang around. I had no fever, chills or flulike symptoms. I had not started physical therapy as yet, and was just waiting daily for signs of my drainage to slow. Finally at the end of week three, my drainage dropped down between fifty to ninety milliliters for the twenty-four-hour period. I thought this would have slowed down sooner. I still could not believe how fatigued I felt. I am such a type-A personality I did not like the patience I needed to have, nor did I like being the patient. But my patience was wearing thin and fatigue is the driver in my life at the moment. This is when you need to let other people help you out. I am so ready to have this suction bulb removed.

This is what I needed to learn, patience. Again a test of trust, as the only peace I knew I would find that could quiet my impatience down was to discover something new about my Maker. His peace surpasses all understanding. I feel so small in comparison to His Omnipresence. I kept saying to myself, *He already knows how this moment and circumstance unfolds. I must wait. Be patient and see what He is going to do with me. It had completely calmed me before, I need to continue my focus on Him.* By the fourth week post-op, my drainage was down to forty-five to sixty milliliters daily. Still no cigar! My surgeon had me see her at the fourth week post-op time frame, because at some point she needed to decide if there was benefit to leaving the drain in and running the risk of infection, or pulling the drain out and risking the chance of swelling and lymphedema. For some people the drain is in two weeks, some shorter, and for some of us longer is necessary. Having twenty-five lymph nodes removed plays a big role in the body's need to redirect traffic, so to speak. Now the body needs to compensate for the sudden increase in fluid. Much like a freeway: when the exit ramp is blocked, the freeway becomes impacted, congested, and traffic slows. Only when the cars that meant to exit find an alternate exit will the traffic begin to resume flow again.

Medical Pearl

The lymphatic system is part of a larger system in the body. The body will notice there has been a change, and it will do all it can to try and compensate for this loss or change.

My drainage was down to forty-five to sixty milliliters in the twenty-four-hour period. With my bulb intact, I headed to Stanford to visit and prayed she will be removing my drain. I would have two appointments: a visit with my surgeon and oncologist. With my doctor, we reviewed all that's going on with my arm, my left breast, and the drainage. I thanked her for preserving the nerves, as I was so pleased to be able to move my arm. My scars were tender and large. I had limitations with how high I could lift my arm up over my head, as well as how long I could keep it up without going into severe cramping or spasms, but I knew I would work hard to gain it all back with exercise and physical therapy.

While her nurse distracted me with conversation, the surgeon pulled my drain out. I never even felt it. I love the little tricks us nurses try to do for our patients to minimize the 'freak-out' of the 'is it going to hurt?' moment. That's what I would call it. They got me! I did not feel a thing. The best part was I got home with a little Band Aid covering my drainage site. She decided to get me started in physical therapy. A referral was placed to the lymphedema-trained therapist in Turlock, close to my home. We agreed I could try swimming again in a few days once the drain site was completely healed over. I was encouraged to continue wearing a compression garment. Something tight to keep the breast swelling down. This was really uncomfortable, much like when your breasts are engorged when you've stopped nursing. Bind the breasts! They are beasts!

A REASONABLE DECISION

My appointment with the oncologist was more supportive of whatever I decided at this time. I suppose if I really needed some medicinal therapy, I am sure they would have strongly advised me to consider it, or certainly made it clear what would happen if I chose otherwise. But in this case, my case, there was no real direction provided. It really is all about the individual lifestyle, mental health, and overall well-being of the patient. What course of treatment a patient would opt for with the exact same diagnosis will vary because of all these factors. However, I had taken notes and made a little grid regarding my options including the trial and the associated risks with each option. As I reviewed all that I understood regarding my options again with him, he concluded it was reasonable to do quarterly diagnostic surveillance monitoring and forgo the immunotherapy and trial at this time. I felt this was a 'benefit' decision also, and it outweighed any unnecessary risks associated with these very powerful medications. He suggested I tried meditation or yoga, something that can distract the mind from worry and pain once again. I mentioned I was engaging in an amazing spiritual walk, and he said that is great also. It was a good day.

Now we shall see what awaits me. It will take some time for the lymphatic detour to occur. But only time will tell. *Only time will tell.* How many times have you heard that in your life? We all have either said it, or we've heard it, or we've had it said to us. Give it time. Time is the answer. In time. It takes time. What a little four letter word, T I M E. Yet, the unforeseen and distant amount of hours, days, months or years it can take, where we finally can say—*Well, there it is.* Closure. *I'm over this hurdle. I'm doing well, I'm moving on. It's in the past and I have healed.* But my favorite would be, *I am cured and cancer-free.* It is all unforeseen to us and surpasses all understanding. It will ALL be revealed in 'due time.'

There is a reason our Lord does not reveal or share too much about our future. For He made our minds the fussiest part of our body. If our every thought is consumed with worry, where is there time for Him? How can we calm ourselves in our heart, mind, and spirit to be thankful and ever present with Him? Being with Him in stillness so He can meet us in the quietness of our souls is the peace I find I need. This is my meditation.

APPRECIATE TODAY – OR – WORRY ABOUT TOMORROW

In July 2016, I enjoyed a three-week vacation to three different states. Our travels were shared with our best friends of over thirty-five years. The four of us enjoyed delicious meals, hikes with captivating sceneries, great conversations and other excursions. With views of the most majestic mountain ranges with their heavenly heights, each gracefully flowing from one snowcapped peak to another. We were able to appreciate their exquisite beauty for miles and miles. It was a very ethereal experience in itself, to be able to witness some of the raw landscaped beauty in this world. Spectacular. Wildlife we had never seen before, water so turquoise-blue that looked refreshing but had temperatures hotter that you can even imagine. There was fun, games, laughter, and the trip ended with a special event of a wedding. Our dear friend's middle son was to be married out in the middle of an expansive meadow which was surrounded by mountain ranges and topped with a heavenly blue sky. *While they were not married in a church, this was most definitely God's Cathedral* I thought. The wedding was full of love and fun. Memories for a lifetime.

In October 2016, we were expecting our fourth grandchild. Another blessing from God. A healthy baby boy. But what if God would have revealed to me what 2017 had in store? Could I have enjoyed the adventure with my friends, the grand beauty of this earth, or appreciated the miracle of birth to its fullest? If I had known the challenges that lay awaiting me, I would have struggled to find peace and joy in all these moments, definitely. The chronic moment-by-moment worry would have been overwhelming in awaiting this challenge. There would be no peace in my immediate future awaiting me.

Spiritual Pearl ~ Seven

I believe God could reveal peace in our future if He wishes to. For some He will show but a glimpse of the future, but only for His purpose. If at all. It's paying attention and appreciating these special moments. These very moments are transforming as I feel Him reveal a peace for me. That is when the Holy Spirit penetrates deeper into our being and the joy and love that follows begins to surpass and defeat the mind's hold on you. Once that racing heart and mind is defeated, then and only then will peace be allowed in. If we can find time to be still, we can experience peace in the stillness of the moment. This is where He will join us for a chat. Sometimes He speaks to us through a loved one's encouraging words or a friend's visit when we least expect it. It may be in the gentle breeze that quietly brushes our neck or cheek as we go about the day. He gives us peace in the stillness of these moments, even when we simply and undistractedly watch the leaves flicker on their branches. If we can appreciate the quiet beauty in that moment, we can feel the peace it can bring with it. That Perfect Peace. Adjusting our eyes and ears to listening more and taking in the beauty that surrounds us, we can experience Him giving us a moment with Him.

CHAPTER FIFTEEN

FIVE AND SIX WEEKS POST-OP

PHYSICAL THERAPY BEGINS AND A FAMILY CRISIS

I was looking forward to starting physical therapy, and my first appointment was about five weeks post-operative. I had been carefully doing some exercises at home as they had encouraged me to do. Some of the exercises I found helpful are included in the next couple of pages.

Entering my fifth week post-op, I tried to take pain one day at a time. Sometimes I found I took three steps forward, other days felt like I took two steps back. The pain continued in the upper arm, much like if someone had an inflated blood pressure cuff on my arm. Inflated just enough to the tightness of its grip, and you could not shake it off once again. The sensations continued to vary. I guess from all I have read at this point, many seem to complain of this: probably it is reasonably normal. I could still wear my wedding band, see the bone in my wrist (ulnar, the bone opposite the thumb side of the hand), bend all my joints (elbow, wrists, and fingers), and see the blood vessels in my hands. These are all good signs and we need to pay attention to these little signs.

But there is a fullness I am noticing in the axilla region that ranges from feeling like a golf ball to just feeling full. I find little mobility in the region, meaning not a soft tissuelike feeling but rather like I was pressing on a plum, with little give. Then there was my deltoid/shoulder cramp which was something I thought would be present for quite some time. But my delay in starting therapy I was sure had to do with the fact my drain was in for four weeks, and my drainage never did get under the twenty milliliters for the twenty-four-hour period. So if the productivity of fluid were continued, the drain could not collect it—this made sense to me. It would take time for the reroute that I mentioned before. I had to give it more time. But it was filling up.

I am so thankful I found a wonderful occupational therapist who was also a certified lymphatic massage therapist so close to my home. Rachel is very knowledgeable in the area of the lymph system and lymphatic massage. My situation was a little different from just experiencing some lymphedema of the arm, as I had the major swelling of my breast associated with my completion surgery. Something she had never seen before. She usually saw breast cancer patients with mastectomies, so this aggravated dependent swelling with a breast intact was new to her. She started taking multiple measurements up the length of my entire arm, beginning with my wrist and ending around my upper arm. This would be important to establish a baseline for comparison purposes in the future for identifying any increase swelling of the arm. Also she was able to properly measure me for a compression garment, or sleeve. After a proper measurement is taken by a professional to give you the size and length to purchase your sleeve, go shop at: www.Lymphdivas.com and search for a garment you prefer. They have many different prints and styles. If you ever wanted to have a tattoo, these sleeves have gorgeous prints for the entire length of the arm. But it is a tattoo I can switch in style and color, or take off any time I want. I purchased two sleeves and they run about $40 to $60 a piece or higher. For compression bras or undergarments, plastic surgeons often refer patients to the website www.marena.com, and again they have many different styles and colors. The cost depends on the style, but can run around $40 to $80 a piece. I had to purchase a few of these, as they encouraged I keep my breast compressed to see if this aided in minimizing the swelling.

Needless to say I had not been very comfortable with my post-op course, not just with my arm but also my breast. Rachel taught me how to gently massage the accessory lymph depots (or basins) areas of my body. This is really important to help the lymphatic system try and establish a new memory and signal or allow the alternate lymphatic cluster zones to help out. This is for the necessary rerouting of fluid, as we discussed before. The largest groupings are found in the neck, armpits, and groin areas. We also have some located directly under our belly button. The massaging of these zones is ever so gentle, as lymph nodes are very delicate and can be injured. Remember they have another job to do other than reroute. They also carry white blood cells, which are responsible for protecting against viruses and bacteria, and they may trap other foreign cells. Hence the gentle pressure, followed by a complete release of that pressure. This massage is repeated five times for all the alternate groupings two to three times daily.

When I have a lymph massage, I can feel the fluid being moved around. Maybe it means the other lymph nodes are kicking in. I know this sounds funny, but the sensation is there and again the physiology of fluid movement under the skin can happen, and maybe the nodes were appreciating the fluid within their region. I had mentioned this to Rachel. She saw the redness in the breast. I mentioned my physicians felt this was most likely a normal probability, although they had not seen it before. All thought it was most likely due to the increase amount of lymph fluid sitting in the breast, which would raise the risk of infection (much like mastitis) being there. And again it made sense. We can physically see the lymph fluid under the skin, as there is a yellow hue to it. If the areas of my breast weren't already red, then they had a yellow hue to them, as did my entire areola. I did not do the 'freak-out,' but a body imagery change for sure. Personal sharing for you women who have had the complete lymph dissection or are considering it for your treatment: I think this is a physiological change and can be a variation of normal. The entire massage treatment was about one hour, and I left with some homework to do until our next visit.

Some exercises that are very helpful and must become a part of your daily routine include:

Physical Therapy Exercises

The Forehead and Pillow Rest: Practicing elevating the effected arm up over your head and resting it on your forehead while lying down, and then laying it behind your head on a pillow. That is tough to do at the start, as cramping like a charley-horse is not uncommon in the deltoid area and arm-pit itself and lateral region (side). Yikes. Most likely, like myself I would have to gently massage this area and it would take a couple minutes to resolve the cramp. The amount of time I can keep it over my head has improved over time. Almost eight months out as I write this, I am successful and the stretch is there. I know my swimming has helped with this. But the cramping does still occur more often than not. I don't know if this will ever completely go away.

The Wall Crawl: With your fingertips on the wall or door, slowly walk them up the wall or door as high as you can tolerate. I challenged myself to do better every time and hold it for a count of ten and repeat it five times daily.

The Chest Cross: Stretching the arm across your chest, keeping your elbow high and touching your other shoulder with your hand. Holding it for a count of ten and repeat.

Scratch Your Back: With one arm reaching back to scratch your upper back with your elbow up, try and meet your fingers of the bad arm behind your back. Fingers reaching up to touch each other. Better yet if you can clasp and unclasp your bra snaps behind your back, hurray! This is an accomplishment.

Doorway Stretch: Every time you go through a doorway, place both hands on each side of the door entry about head height. Your feet should be one in front of the other as if you were getting ready to kneel down (but don't kneel), then gently press your upper body through the doorway. Gently feeling the stretch in the upper chest and axillary area. Cramping usually will occur. Stop as you need to and repeat this. Anytime we can stretch the underarm area gently is good.

Exercise is great for the arm whenever you can. But in the beginning everything is really fragile and we must be ginger at first. Take it slow and believe me, it is s-l-o-w. But I will not give up and I'm confident I will regain some form of normalcy soon, I hope.

THE FAMILY CRISIS

While I was in my very first session of massage therapy, I had my cell phone on silent. When I returned to my car after therapy, I noticed I had five missed calls, all from my husband who was working from home. It was the Friday after Mother's Day. He asked me to call him as soon as possible and I did. He informed me his mother, who lives a block up from us, had been taken to the hospital and was in a coma. His mother had made plans to go out to lunch with some old friends of many years and her daughter. But she did not answer her door when her friends and daughter had arrived. Her daughter had just spoken to her on the phone two hours prior. When her daughter let herself in, she found her mother lying face down on the floor in her bathroom. She had managed to lie down and propped her head gently on a folded towel. My thought was she must have experienced a very bad headache so she placed a towel under her head and lay down.

He had been asked about her Advanced Directive so I texted it to him, as I had all her medical information in a file on my phone. Thank you God for the gift of organization! We had completed her Advanced Directive just earlier this year. I rushed to the hospital thirty minutes away, only to find my husband very distressed about his mother as was I. He said he was sitting at our dining room table working when out of the front widow, he saw the ambulance with lights flashing turn the corner. He got a pit in his stomach and went out to see where it stopped—it was at his mother's. We can see her garage doors from our house and sure enough that was where it stopped. He ran down the street, and emergency medical systems were initiated. Then he made his way to the hospital.

Without belaboring the details, she had a massive brain hemorrhage that she would not recover from. The physicians said she was sure to pass within a matter of hours to a day. My husband and his sister contacted the remaining siblings to fill them in the shocking event, and it was decided to initiate a breathing machine to keep her breathing until the remainder of the family could fly in to say their goodbyes. The remaining siblings were coming from all over the country. They would all be able to arrive by the following night. So the plan was to keep her on life support until everyone had arrived. They could say their goodbyes, and then they would discontinue the breathing machine and let her naturally pass, but keep her as comfortable as possible. The physicians agreed with the plan.

The reason I am choosing to share this part of our life with you is there were a couple very spiritual moments that occurred. It was a powerful family moment that many of you may have already experienced. The death of a loved one. Never fun to go through, but when it is unexpected and over, there is no time to prepare for goodbyes. The siblings all arrived safely the following evening, on Saturday. There was a wide range of emotions as you would expect for our beloved matriarch. We had planned to congregate in the hospital chapel once everyone had arrived, to be able to prepare everyone for what they were about to see. We also wanted to have a moment of silence and prayer before we made our way to her room, for most likely what would be our last visit.

Holy Spirit Moment ~ Six

My husband had just returned from spending time in her room and the chaplain stopped him in the hallway and handed him a scripture pamphlet. He told my husband he had prayed over his mother earlier and read her some scripture. He then recommended my husband continue to pray with her and start with the first scripture outlined in the handout. So my husband took the handout and we all walked into the chapel. There were about sixteen or so of us. I suggested to my husband we prepare everyone for the visual impact her apparent state would be. She was unresponsive, pale, and frail in appearance. They would hear breathing machine noise, beeping noises, and see different tubes including one in her mouth. Also they could notice some involuntary movements that might seem like she was responding, but this can occur and in this case did not mean recovery was hopeful. This would be a very sad, uncomfortable, and unforgettable last vision of our sweet happy Mema. Anyone who wanted to say their goodbyes could, and the remainder of us would be waiting in the chapel for hugs and support.

So we all stood in a circle holding hands. Some of us were practicing Christians and some family members were not believers. But all showed respect and love during this time. So my husband started by saying how he had just seen the chaplain who handed him a pamphlet with scripture suggestions and recommended he start with the very first one in the pamphlet. He then proceeded and read the very first scripture passage the chaplain had recommended:

"Be still and know that I am God; I will be exalted among the nations, I will be exalted in the earth. The Lord Almighty is with us; the God of Jacob is our fortress,"

PSALM 46:10–11

Then my husband continued, "You are all aware of what Lita has been going through. What is so amazing here is this was the chaplain's encouragement for scripture reading to be shared, and it is the exact scripture I would recite in the middle of the night when I would awaken with worry about Lita. This is the presence of the Holy Spirit with this family right now." My husband shared with me later he could not believe this was merely a coincidence. No, this was confirmation once again that the Holy Spirit is near and the Lord is even nearer. Amongst us at that very moment. He finished with his prayer and we opened it up for anyone to say whatever they wanted to say. His brother prayed and then my daughter said some words. Then another scripture was read by my nephew;

"The Lord is near. Do not be anxious about anything, but in every situation, by prayer and petition, with thanksgiving, present your requests to God. And the peace of God, which transcends all understanding, will guard your hearts and minds in Christ Jesus,"

PHIL 4:5–7. *NIV*

No coincidences here either, as this was the exact scripture I would recite to myself in the middle of the night when I would awaken with worry, or my heart be racing. As I have stated in the beginning of this book. The Holy Spirit is near. Coincidence that both my husband's and my favorite 'go to' verses are recited here tonight? I know they are strong verses for situations like these, but I'll stick with the Holy Spirit is near. Again.

Later that night, after we had all said our goodbyes, my daughter shared with me that she experienced another vision while in deep prayer in the chapel. We were all standing in a circle holding hands and in prayer when she had a vision of Jesus with outstretched arms standing in the midst of our family circle. He was cloaked in a whiter-than-white gown. He appeared exactly the way He had appeared to her while I was undergoing surgery. She had tears streaming down her face when she told me. The power of this vivid vision so clearly overwhelmed her. We knew our precious Mema would be in heaven, for once again Jesus was present amongst us and He made Himself visible to her. We did not have any doubts regarding her faith, as she had mentioned before she believed in God. I noticed she was trying to spend some time in the Word lately, as I saw her reading it when I would swing by for a quick visit.

When we struggle with a challenge or stressor of any sort, including loss, they can build strength and character for us to move forward in a healthy manner. It's a fact of life, and I think the more we love someone, the longer the heart will ache. Another trial in life where the Lord says, *I am preparing your character so you may find strength to persevere.* And when we persevere, He knows this renders hope. And the best thing about hope is that it came from God and is always good. Character building from trials makes us stronger and is necessary. It was an extremely emotional and exhausting evening to say the least. Most of the family had all gone to their respective lodging for the night. The breathing machine was discontinued, and Mema continued to breathe shallowly for the next day.

We had been to the hospital on Sunday off and on all day and kept in touch with the nursing staff throughout the night. Monday morning I headed to the hospital. My brother-in-law, Tom, was staying with us, and he mentioned to me the nurse had called and said her breathing was really labored now. I said, "We have to go now," but he needed to shower as he had been with her several hours during the night. So he and my husband were going to come in a separate car, just five minutes behind me, and I left for the hospital. When I arrived at her room, two nurses were standing there documenting things. Walking through the door I asked, "What is going on?" They said she had just expired. I knew the time was very near, but I just missed being with her. The reality hit me: this sweet mother-in-law of mine was gone. I started to cry and I asked if I could have a moment with her. I recited the Lord's Prayer and whispered in her ear, "You go be with your groom." She had been missing her husband so much for these past seven years. Within the past year she had felt his presence at night with her. 'He felt close,' she had said. Then I called my husband, who had just arrived in the parking lot of the hospital and was heading up. She was gone. Just like that—gone. However, she arrives in heaven exactly on schedule.

The next few days were busy with discussion and initial arrangements. The decision was made to do a Celebration of Life for her in mid-August. We had nieces and nephews in college, then there was police academy training starting, new jobs, and other commitments that absolutely could not be changed. Like holding two-, one-week camp sessions for underprivileged kids on my brother-in-law's property in North Carolina, which he and my sister-in-law run with other family members helping out. We had to postpone it. We wanted the entire family to be able to attend. She deserved the best. So an August date was set to celebrate this gracious lady. I was so blessed with my in-laws. I know she felt the love from her family, because she gave love freely. We had just shared an amazing Mother's Day with her. She was the happiest and most relaxed I had ever seen her. She had celebrated with my husband and our family on Saturday with a BBQ and all the grandkids and four of her great-grandchildren were here. Then her daughter's family who was local celebrated with her on Sunday. She was treated very special the entire weekend, and had really enjoyed every event. The remaining siblings had called to send their Best-Mom-Ever wishes. When we spoke about it later in the hospital while she was in a coma, we agreed something was different about her. She was exuberantly happy. Five days later she had a massive stroke, and now is with Our Creator. She was honored with a beautiful Celebration of Life service and she would have been very pleased had she been sitting in the front row of the audience. I am sure she was there smiling and blushing about all the wonderful things said about her, as she took in the aroma of all the exquisite flowers.

How wonderful to have lived a love-filled life; she made it easy to put a eulogy together.

SIX WEEKS POST-OP, REDNESS SPREADING

The following morning, Tuesday, I decided to go swimming after being cleared for this. This was my very first swim after my complete axillary surgery. I was really looking forward to this day. But I noticed my breast was even redder than the day prior and after my physical therapy (PT) appointment. I had no itching, aches or pains, fever or chills. I went swimming anyway and wore my swim shirt. I always wear an SPF swim shirt now, no matter what time of day I chose to swim. I wore sunscreen also, and I was swimming at 7:30 in the morning. I had a decent workout. I took it easy. I swam about a mile. Which is about sixty-four laps in a twenty-five-meter pool. I did not swim them all at once, doing my usual sets instead and resting when I needed to.

It was so therapeutic. Again I was in my underwater world and enjoying the serenity and simplicity of my swim. When you exercise you feel like you have some control of your own destiny regarding recovery. And we do. We must exercise the arm and regain strength in the muscles. Carefully though, so as to not add insult to the injury. Swimming aids in attending to my mental well-being, which is a must when we are dealing with cancer, and more so now that I am mourning the loss of a loved one. Again whether meditation, yoga, or another hobby, distraction from an ongoing challenge is vital to our mental wellness. Swimming has an added benefit: it is a natural compression exercise for the arm. So this aids in promoting lymph fluid movement with compression results all in one. I don't know how my arm will respond until I test it. So I give it a little push at a time.

Over the next couple days my breast and chest became more reddish in color. With a confluent rash, I thought I noted it to be spreading. Whatever 'it' was, it was spreading upward into my upper chest area and around my breast. I thought possibly an infection just under the skin called cellulitis. I had made a follow-up appointment with my local surgeon, and after examination she advised me to restart antibiotic therapy with two different kind of antibiotics. The same antibiotics we would treat woman with mastitis. I have been on so many antibiotics throughout the past eight months. It gets old, but what else are we going to do with these symptoms. I cannot let myself get frustrated and need to continue to pay attention to my symptoms. Ignorance is not bliss, and it is my job for now. It is also important that we stay compliant as to the plan laid out by our physicians, as this helps with evaluating the results so they may ascertain the next course of action if the current plan renders unsatisfactory results.

She wanted to see me back in late September for recheck breast exam and a breast ultrasound, as well as tomographic mammogram or 3D mammogram. She had not seen this level of lymphedema in a breast like I was experiencing, as her patients have usually undergone a mastectomy. But again the physiology of this made sense. The trick with all the additional lymph fluid stagnant within the breast tissue is to prevent mastitis from occurring and making sure we can get it under control. Antibiotics should help, so we will see. I started the fourteen days of therapy with two different medications.

I had another physical therapy session with my lymphatic specialist about three days after my swim, and about five days from my last lymph massage therapy session. We discussed the changes in my left breast and my skins continued rashlike appearance. My areola was still yellow in hue. I underwent a full hour of lymphatic massage therapy. She does such a great job with light massage of the arm and then the light compression to the other lymphatic zones to promote stimulation. This allows them some activation to get them working and again aiding in the rerouting of fluid, as I have mentioned. I am aware of the sensation of fluid working its way around under the skin. It felt really good and I could feel it was shifting and the tissue softening once therapy is complete.

But for a day or two after my massage, I did note some increase in discomfort. I suspect with any physical therapy, post-discomfort from the workout must be expected. The therapist is not only working on getting the fluid moving, but also on stretching the arm, especially the underside of the arm. That is where I note the greatest sensation of fullness, tightness, and limitation. Whether it is from the fluid collection, scarring from the webbing, or just interstitial swelling I do not know. But one complication to pay attention to is the development of **axillary web syndrome (AWS)**, also known as webbing or cording. This can vary in degrees of pain and range from person to person with the extent of involvement varying also. This sometimes develops as a possible side effect of sentinel lymph node biopsy (SLNB) or axillary lymph node dissection (ALND) surgeries. This may occur within several days, weeks, or in some cases even months after surgery. Scar tissue from the surgery to the axillary area may contribute to the discomfort of tightness and pain. It can be excruciating, and I think I have a high pain tolerance.

If you develop axillary webbing, you will often be able to see or feel a web of thin to thick ropelike structures under the skin of the inner arm. Often you will notice them when you raise your arm up shoulder level or above your head. Sometimes they are not visible, but you experience sensations of pain and tightening, and this may indicate they are indeed there. Massaging and stretching these areas out is very important, and it needs to be ongoing in our therapy. I could feel the cords; some were larger in diameter than others. The discomfort and tightening varied from day to day with me. But the sensation began in my underarm area and extended to my elbow. I could palpate it with my fingers from my upper inner arm, all the way down to my wrist at times. When they are stretched or massaged, it definitely created some intense discomfort for me. At times it is very difficult to keep my arm raised above my head for a length of time without experiencing pain or that Charley-horse-like cramping. Physical pain is fatiguing.

As with any surgery, internal scarring can create similar issues. This is a side effect, but with the extent of complete lymph node dissection, I would estimate it occurs more often than not. Whether it is always diagnosed is a different subject. But if the syndrome is noted, it should be addressed with a lymphedema therapist. Stretching and trying to release them is important for mobility. I do believe they can be more noticeable at times as I am bothered by them more often and more intensely than not. But the massage therapy to these areas reminds me, they are very much there and I need to continue with my homework to work through them, to promote flexibility. We must fight through the pain.

Within the next day, I noted the redness in my chest area and swelling in my breast is continuing. The process of the rerouting of lymph fluid is significant and can vary in the time it takes for the body to initiate this on its own. I feel I am still not there. The areas of redness under my skin extends from my upper chest and breast to just below my breast in the upper abdomen and are continuing to spread. I continued with my antibiotics and have only a few days left. The redness of the rash has never subsided. In fact, after my massage therapy session, I noted it became worse and continued to spread in more rapid pace. I still remain asymptomatic in other areas. Again no fever, chills, flulike symptoms, or anything that I was actually concerned with. But what was I going to do now? I took pictures of my areas of concern and through my medical patient portal, I emailed my surgeon at Stanford. She advised I just continue the antibiotics longer. Another ten days of them, so I did.

Obviously recovering isn't the only thing going on in life. We had celebrated more family birthdays, and thank goodness for distractions. What joy I find in having my family over for something as simple as a BBQ. The grandkids running all over the house. Chatter in the air with laughing and sometimes crying. Then all the cuddles and love the little cousins give each other and me! I can't tell you how many times they wanted to see 'my ball' when it was attached to me, or kiss my Boo-Boo! They knew I had something going on. My oldest granddaughter, who just turned six, was very cautious around me and she would watch me to see if I smiled or laughed. She often knew if I wasn't feeling well. I noticed she was more herself when she thought I was more myself. She was worrying about me. Precious Karrington. These little ones pay attention to what is going on around them, and they worry—but don't know how to express it. I also love that my family knows how to pitch in when I don't even ask. All of them, my son-in-law's too. A happy distraction is welcomed!

This is when I say: *before I bring my needs, I will bring my praise.*

CHAPTER SIXTEEN

SEVEN TO TEN WEEKS POST-OP

SEVEN TO EIGHT WEEKS POST-OP

Time seems to go by slowly with the day-to-day, same ole same ole discomfort. It is truly exhausting. I am exhausted, no energy, but I try and just keep going about my day. As for my arm, progress seems at a snail's pace. The discomfort continues. There are times when I feel no bothersome sensations at all, but only for a few minutes at a time. Very hard to describe, I cannot count on what is in store for me in regards to my arm on a day-to-day basis. Every day is the same, though I can count on something! I can say right now "I am so over this," but the reality is my arm may never be completely normal again. Another couple of weeks have passed and I am now on another round of antibiotic treatment and more tired than usual. There just does not seem to be noticeable improvement from antibiotics with the redness. It seems to be spreading gradually and steadily. It really is the weirdest thing. It has almost reached my collar bone, and down to my belly button in what seemed to be overnight. No signs of it stopping. My husband is heading out of town for three days on business, and will be about three hours away by car. I told him to go as it was a team-building getaway, and reassured him I would be fine. I had a friend coming from out of town the following day to visit and go to lunch. I would call him if I needed him. So off he went.

A COMPLICATION

My best friend Peggy arrived midmorning and we were going to have a nice lunch out. We have been friends since we were fifteen. We made small talk and I filled her in on my health update. We know each other very well, to say the least. I mentioned to her something was just not sitting right with me. My gut was once again saying something else must be going on. It kept gnawing at me and she knows from past experiences that my gut is usually right. I think most times when our gut just doesn't sit well that it is the Holy Spirit trying to get our attention, aside from Him saying, "Lita, something IS wrong, so go take care of it." We need to listen to that little voice inside of us and not doubt it so much. We have all heard it at one time or another, but paying attention to it and trusting it is a different story. We went to also pick up her mother and off to lunch we went. At the end of lunch, she said to me, "Lita, if you think something is not quite right, listen to your gut and do what you think you need to do." After about a two-hour lunch, we said our good-byes.

After she drove away, I found myself driving to the emergency room. I parked in the visitor's parking lot and sat in my car for thirty-five minutes thinking, *Should I or shouldn't I?* I was trying to decide if I should walk into this emergency room, which has access to the same medical records system as my physicians at Stanford, or drive to the other emergency room, because that was where my local breast surgeon had privileges. I texted my husband and we agreed I would walk into the emergency room. It was three-thirty in the afternoon. I did not let anyone else know, but I promised I would update him.

So after waiting thirty-five minutes in my car, I was dreading it but I walked into the ER waiting room. I was expecting to see a room full of people, but there was not a single person inside waiting. Not a soul around, except for the staff person behind the counter. I could not believe it.

Immediately I said, *"Holy Spirit are you here with me?"* This room is cleared out, and it is one of the busiest emergency rooms in town. When have you EVER walked into an ER and no one else was there waiting? I walked right up to the desk and she took the usual information which included: why are you visiting us today? Well, I am visiting you because... blah-blah-blah. I mentioned my recent history with my surgery and that this redness was spreading across my chest and up my neck and down my abdomen, blah-blah-blah. The nurse came, got me, and into the exam room I went.

There was the visit from the ER doctor, and at length we discussed my symptoms. This included the fact my drain had been removed only 4 weeks prior, and the redness that continued to spread over my midsection and breast clear up to my collarbone. I was asked by three physicians who saw me if I had undergone 'radiation treatment' to my chest. That is how red and raw it looked. Other than it being slightly warm to the touch, I had no other symptoms. The symptoms that remained consistent were feeling extremely fatigued, and it was spreading steadily. Feeling exhausted was a daily reality. My vital signs were taken, and I requested the physician call my surgeon at Stanford, which he gladly did. He was able to get a hold of her, they spoke, and a plan was outlined. We needed to access what was going on under my axillary region. This was definitely going to postpone my vacation planned for Maui at the end of the month. Didn't I mention we were going to Maui? Well, we aren't going now. I just had another 'gut' feeling about needing to reschedule this trip.

My husband had texted my girls on what was going on and before I knew it, my oldest daughter, Lindsay, and my mother were walking in to be with me. They decided no one should be sitting in an ER alone. Who likes waiting in an ER? No one that I can think of, not me for sure! One thing I know for sure is I am still not liking this whole patient thing. The decision was made to start an IV and some intravenous antibiotics. Two very powerful and broad spectrum antibiotics. Blood cultures were done to see if I had a systemic blood infection or sepsis going on. With this type of surgery, I had a new allergy warning; also, nothing could be done in or on my left arm. This leaves only my right arm to take all the blood pressures, shots, IVs, and blood cultures. I hope my one little vein in my hand can hang in there through all this. An axillary ultrasound was done about eight-thirty that night and it was concluded that I had a fluid pocket under my arm. Being a sonographer myself, I could tell it did not appear like a simple collection of fluid. Which would have been lymphatic fluid. But instead, to me it appeared to be moderate in size, with septate-like appearance within it (meaning compartmentlike appearance), and the echogenicity within the pocket seemed consistent with a hematoma, which is a blood-filled pocket. This finding sheds light on my discomfort, fatigue, and hmmm. All would be revealed when the drain most likely would be reinserted sometime tomorrow. That was the plan for now.

After a couple doses of IV antibiotics, cultures, and the sonogram being done, I went home for the night. My insurance carrier computer was down, supposedly, so obtaining authorization to actually admit me to the hospital was out. The ER physician gave me the following options: stay and take chances absorbing the bill or wait until we can get approval tomorrow morning first thing. Well, let me think about this one! He also assured me that once the insurance authorization for hospitalization was approved, he would call me and likely want to admit me first thing in the morning. I would be receiving more IV antibiotics, the possibility of a drain reinsertion was looming but probable. Routine blood work and blood cultures were to be continued as per request of my surgeon at Stanford, and the two physicians would stay in touch. Well, I guess my gut was right again. I left the hospital ER around 10:00 PM that night. I spoke with my husband, who was committed into coming home and safely did so about 12:45 AM. Bless his heart, and thank you God for getting him home safe at that hour. Hospitalization would be the next reality awaiting me tomorrow morning, and who knows for how long. But it was time for answers and I was ready to hear them.

HOSPITALIZATION AND DRAIN REINSERTION

I received the call around 9:30 AM the next morning and was promptly admitted to the hospital upon arrival. Thank goodness I was able to secure a private room. I was not feeling well enough to have any activity coming or going on around me. The previously mentioned plan was to be executed. I wasn't sure if the attempt would be to simply drain the area in question or reinsert the new drain, with a plan of leaving it in. Who knows for how long I would need it in place. Either way it was discouraging for me. A setback I thought for sure. How do you not get discouraged when you have been doing everything expected of you, stayed compliant in post-op instructions trying to recover and then a complication? And you know what they say, doctors are the worst patients. Again, I find myself vulnerable and anxious with so much out of my control. I am truly exhausted, so you get the picture, but at the same time needing resolution to this mysterious symptom. Within my arsenal of notes and scripture, I lean on knowing My Lord is near. I began reciting my Philippians 4:5–7 over and over. What hurdles will I have in store for me next? God knows and He will guard my heart and mind through Christ Jesus. He was preparing me for something. I didn't know what. By the way, still no thought of writing this book; it was on His mind, not mine.

For those of you hospitalized before, the usual routine chaos ensued. You do not relax or sleep well while in a hospital. They knew I was a nurse practitioner. I was speaking the medical language too easily and they asked if I was a nurse, so I told them. This may have helped with getting a private room allocated. But also the hospital census was low, which means patient admittance was low. This actually may have helped me out more. Who really knows, maybe they thought I would be infectious and needed to isolate me. Either way, I was glad I had the medical knowledge I had. I knew what questions to ask. I was my own advocate. I don't know if the general population knows that they can be assigned a patient advocate or translator if they don't understand what the staff or doctor is trying to explain regarding their care. This is one of our rights as patients. This is one of those situations when I am glad I know what I know, because I need to know. You know?

I was scheduled for my repeat ultrasound with guidance to place the new pigtail drain back in the axillary area late in the afternoon. The sonogram guidance allows the radiologist to see exactly where the best placement for the drain tubing to be, to allow drainage of the most fluid. Sometimes there are multiple pockets or septums (compartments) that keep pockets

of fluid separated, requiring more than one drain to be placed. I was fortunate the ultrasound showed a more complex form of fluid, consistent with
a collection of blood, and only one drain was placed. The area of concern
appeared to have multiple septate (dividers) within the entire blood-filled
pocket. Like I suspected the night before. But he decided most likely those
smaller pockets would reabsorb eventually. They gave me a little sedation,
the drain was placed for optimum resolution for the size collection of blood.
Hopefully, it will adequately resolve the issue. I was able to have a conversation with the radiologist during the procedure. He confirmed as the output
began to drain that it was indeed blood. He did a culture on the fluid to
ensure there was no infection present within the wound.

So back to my room I went, my new drain intact and doing what it was
supposed to do—draining. For the next three days I had blood work twice
daily. Blood cultures were drawn twice daily to check for any systemic infectious process. It would take a full seven days to get an accurate result from
these blood cultures. I had intravenous infusion going on all day, with two
very potent antibiotics administered twice daily. I think the diagnosis was
infection in the skin or cellulitis. But I never had a fever, which usually goes
with it. No other symptoms. Just this raging red angry skin rash that was
spreading. Hopefully the powerful antibiotics would aid in resolving this
confluent rash, which at first seemed to be holding steady.

For the first day or two my output of blood was steady, slowing by the
third day. I was tired. My labs indicated I was anemic, as my hemoglobin
had dropped almost six points, but not low enough for a blood transfusion,
which is a blessing. I had lost just under one pint of blood total. I was so
ready to go home and crawl into my own bed with my own real pillow and
fall asleep for a week! Don't you wish we could really do that sometime?
Even a good long nap—maybe only for three days—I would welcome and it
is all I really needed. Then while I'm napping, the whole world just needs to
stop so I could catch up.

There may have been a very slight change in the redness on my body; at
least it wasn't getting worse, which was a positive sign. It had stopped spreading. Maybe it was starting to respond to the antibiotics and once the results
of my cultures returned negative, they could release me. The preliminary

report for the blood cultures had been negative and I was not expecting them to change. Discharge instructions were reviewed; I was to continue and complete the course of antibiotics, keep track of my drainage output, and follow up with my surgeon at Stanford on the following Wednesday. I was discharged the day before Father's Day. I was supposed to have a BBQ at my home for all the men in our life, but instead plans got changed to my daughter's home. They all spoiled me that night. It was a delicious meal, and I relished in my squishes from my little grandchildren. It was so good to be home, even with my new friend intact, 'my ball.' I received my Boo-Boo kisses and squishes once again. A happy distraction again, and welcomed.

NINE TO TEN WEEKS POST-OP

What happened? I had a follow-up appointment with my surgeon at Stanford in several days, which would place me around ten weeks post-op. I was continuing with more antibiotics and minding my drainage. Over the next several days the redness of my chest and abdomen was continuing to improve but certainly was not gone. My breast was unchanged, very heavy, large, with redness in areas, and with notable lymph fluid within it. This was extremely frustrating. As for my arm, I continued with pain off and on. Sometimes I felt like I was just a mess. All the sensations continued to come and go, and the intensity had not eased up. But I could still wear my wedding band, see my wrist bones, veins in my hand, and move all my joints. I had the same challenge having the suction drainage bulb again, with showering, dressing, etc. It is mid-June, and all this medical journey began with the initial diagnosis in January. No wonder I was tired. How much longer was this all going to take? Patience was at my door—again.

So during the next several days that followed I started to do some research on skin/dermal reaction as blood seeps slowly into it, but without any form of insult or injury. I formulated my own medical/physiological opinion, without obtaining the opinion of any physician I have surrendered my care to while writing this. Whether I am correct or not, I believe only when the hematoma was able to have an alternate escape route—meaning to be drained out (instead of seeping under the skin to disperse itself) and possibly the antibiotics—was there going to be any resolution to my skin's angry redness. Antibiotics alone did not seem to resolve the issue. So to me this meant one thing: the blood was seeping out from the pocket where it had collected and into the surrounding tissue and surface of the skin. This was the huge, maybe only, contributing factor for the slow spread of extreme redness across my body. I had not experienced a single physician who had ever seen the extent of the redness that I was exhibiting. And as I mentioned, the emergency room physicians and hospitalist all asked if I had undergone radiation treatment to my chest area, which I was pretty sure I would remember if I had. That was how raw, red and angry it appeared, but it never hurt. Any lab work that had been done, or vital sign that had been taken, could reveal or aid in offering even a hint for a diagnosis. There was no straight answer to why this had occurred. There was no infection; it wasn't even a true cellulitis, but we needed a diagnosis that would include an axillary hematoma.

In brief, I wanted to include some explanation for this potential setback, to educate anyone undergoing this surgery how to watch for similar signs as I have fully explained. I've tried to include a simple understanding of this event. These symptoms and everything I just shared with you may sound familiar to some of you reading this. I know I can't possibly be the only one who has undergone a complete axillary dissection surgery that has developed a large hematoma that needed draining. The skin reaction, if any, and the extent of it, probably varies from person to person with this postsurgical setback. The amount of redness, like being dipped in cherry jello, that I experienced may have been fueled by the physical therapy massage to the area on two separate occasions and only three days apart. I had also been walking, swimming, and possibly gravity along with the fact the blood was already pooling in the area may have exaggerated the entire event to what it evolved into. Doesn't this all make sense?

I believe my lymph/immune system was showing me firsthand how it worked. When an accumulation of blood has filled a contained area, with an increase in pressure evolving, a hematoma will form. If the hematoma is not encased (like that of an unruptured hemorrhagic ovarian cyst), it will eventually find a way and begin to seep into other areas of least resistance—if it can. In my case, it found a way. Once the axillary pocket was filled with blood and the pressure had built up enough, hence the 'plum' like fullness, the blood began to overflow or relocate under other areas of my skin. It had spread to my collarbone, my left side, and across my upper abdomen above my belly button. Yes, dipped in cherry jello!

The blood that had pooled (under my arm) and now was overflowing and being absorbed under the skin surface was spreading steadily. It would not be stopped. It was moving, just as it is supposed to do, and it will continue to travel to the areas where the accessory lymph basins could help it be flushed from the body for resolution. Since majority of my lymph nodes were removed under my left arm, it was rerouting itself. Yay! Way to figure it out, body! Remember, every area of our skin has lymph node drainage sites, and I believe this is what it was trying to do. Rerouting was just witnessed with a color chart of 'cherry jello,' and in the form of red rash moving slowly across my body. It was heading up towards my collarbone, where a collection of lymph pearls are, and extended towards my belly button, where another cluster of nodes and filtering site lies. Isn't our bodies design amazing? Even Dr. Francis Collins, the geneticist, was amazed at the complexities of the genetic makeup of the human body, which took him a decade of dedicated work, to which He credits God for His masterful design. Read the book; it has interesting scientific facts.

There is a difference in the reaction of the skin when we experience a bruise as opposed to what has happened to me. Usually with a bruise there has been trauma, usually from an injury, whether it be a surface injury or a deeper injury, and blood does seep under the skin with this also. Aside from the seriousness of the injury (lacerations or broken bones), the surface of the skin eventually proceeds through a normal sequence of skin color change from the injured or dependent area. We have all seen a bruise change colors as healing ensues. If it is a surface injury, the blood from the ruptured capillaries (small blood vessels) near the skin surface escapes by leaking out under the skin. When there is no other place for it to go the blood gets trapped, forming a red or purplish mark that is tender to touch.

It becomes a bruise. The bruise eventually gets reabsorbed, usually with the help of the lymph system.

Following an injury, the blood that has infused itself into the tissue will first appear reddish in color, reflecting the color of blood under the skin. By one or two days, the reddish iron from the blood undergoes a change and the bruise will change from reddish to blue or purple, then on to yellowish-green. From one change of color to the next, the healing and repair continues, until finally the skin returns to its normal color. Sometimes you can tell how long ago an injury occurred from its color stage to the surface of the skin. The tenderness is greatest at beginning of the trauma. But over time, as it goes through the healing process, the tenderness improves gradually as new tissue/capillary repair is underway. Once again, I am amazed how perfectly designed we are and how the body tries to heal.

So when there is no injury or blow to cause this bruiselike reaction, the blood will seep slowly under the skin, possibly cause a dermal response that includes inflammation, redness, and rash like I experienced. There is no tenderness as with a bruise. It can even appear like an allergic reaction. And as the blood continues to move through and under the skin, the reaction occurs. Since no vesicular (vessel or capillaries) damage had been done, and no impact or injury was sustained, the skin will react to the blood cells within it and often appear inflamed and red, until the body can break it down and reabsorb what should not be there to begin with. It may feel warmer in areas, and in my case this was not caused by an infectious process, just physiological response. And the color will not go through the stages of change like that of a bruise; the redness will very, very gradually disappear. This is when the immune system will start to kick in, as I witnessed. It all makes sense. A setback for sure, the frustration is real, and fatigue will continue.

I could feel the discomfort in this change. The pressure under the arm is the hardest to evaluate as to what is 'normal' and what needs to be 'checked out.' Because the post-op instructions do say that if you feel increase in pressure under the arm, let them know. I think the discomfort or pressure feeling is all relative to the pain tolerance level each of us has. My level of discomfort may be your level of excruciating pain, or vice versa! I was very uncomfortable, but then I thought I should expect to be—with this type of surgery. I probably would have tolerated it even longer had there not been the growing redness and slight warmth to my skin. It was the rapid spreading that got my attention, as I didn't sense it was going to stop. It walked me into the ER.

TEN WEEKS POST-OP

So it was June 21st and I was off to my appointment with my cutaneous oncology surgeon at Stanford. I was looking forward to seeing her. We chatted about the past week's event and I was thankful she was able to provide instruction to the ER physicians in my hometown. She accessed my wound, which was healing nicely. She noted the drainage of blood was darker in color and minimal. Both are expected and the volume was under twenty milliliters. She decided to do an axillary sonogram in the office before she pulled the drain, for comparison with the current size of the hematoma. As she scanned the area in question, we all noticed there had definitely been a change. The hematoma was smaller in size. Actually, it was less than half of the size it had been. The reinsertion of the drain had helped, and the pocket of blood was smaller and stable. So in my opinion, the seeping of blood under the skin would stop. The drain was removed without incident, and we were all confident the remainder of the blood pocket would take care of itself. In due time.

As we concluded the appointment, the plan was for some healing time. We did not want to get this bleeding started up again, and there was no way of knowing how it started to begin with. So there would be no physical therapy and no swimming laps until she could reevaluate my condition in four weeks. I continued with the antibiotics and made another appointment four weeks out. My surveillance follow-up included a second set of brain MRI and PET scan, which were scheduled for July as well. I was tired. I was frustrated. I was human.

FAMILY VACATION AT ALTITUDE OF 6,500 FT.

The next four weeks felt like a setback to me, but I tried to make the best of it. I was exhausted and frustrated as mentioned. We had a family vacation coming up at the end of June, renting a cabin at a beautiful lake only an hour and a half away. We went through the process of cancelling our trip to Maui, so this was an alternative plan to spend time with the kids and grandkids. This would be my first attempt at traveling to an elevation that may cause an issue with my arm. The lake is at an elevation of 6,500 feet. The lymphedema instructions encouraged us to wear a compression sleeve when flying, or with any altitude change, and everyone is different. So I had to see how this would affect my arm.

Medical Pearl

Anytime a significant change in elevation or extreme temperature may occur, wearing a compression sleeve would be a preventative measure in minimizing any potential swelling of the arm.

I did not put my sleeve on as we drove up to the lake, but I had brought it with me. I was doing fine right up to about an altitude of 2,500 feet. So I slipped my sleeve on while we were driving. This was all still so new to me. I noticed my arm in general was beginning to ache, with a gripping discomfort around my upper arm, with a sensation of burning that radiated to the elbow. I had felt this before off and on this entire recovery. So I took acetaminophen 1,500 mg, or three Tylenols. This did help take the edge off the discomfort. When we arrived at the cabin, all seemed to be the same regarding the ache within my left arm; it hadn't improved, but had not become worse. I had no swelling of the wrist, hands or fingers, which I was paying close attention to. So we unpacked (my husband did), and slowly the family began to arrive.

I would wear my sleeve throughout the day, taking it off only if I needed a breather from it. They were so binding and tight. Very uncomfortable to wear, let alone having to wear it all day long. But I did what needed to be done. Anything to prevent lymphedema from occurring. I did not wear it at night, as this wasn't a good idea. The compression was so tight that if we fell asleep with our arm bent in this garment, we would probably awaken with swelling of the wrists, hand, and fingers. The additional pressure on the nerves throughout the night might contribute to damaging them. There may be some instances in which the physician will instruct otherwise, as case by case scenarios are different. **But in general, wearing a sleeve compression garment at night is not advised.**

I made sure I did not carry anything on this trip; loading and unloading any beach paraphernalia, etc. was left to someone else. I was able to wade in the lake and entertain my grandchildren to a certain extent. Using only one arm was confining. I really couldn't say if wearing the sleeve really helped. Maybe it was helping in a way I wouldn't really notice, physiologically—at the cellular level. The ache continued whether I was wearing it or not. I erred on the side of wearing it at this elevation. I concluded that my body was going to notice when twenty-five lymph nodes were missing, as their prior role maintained circulatory stability. Especially at this elevation. I reminded myself that I had a history of melanoma stage III, with 'history' being used as past tense. This daily discomfort was my new normal as my recovery continued. I felt good about my decision for the completion surgery even with this pain, but it remained a gradual process adjusting to the appearance of my body and scars. It was a solid choice and possibly life-saving, or therapeutic treatment for me. But when the intensity of pain is significant, one cannot help get frustrated with the situation. Some of you may be asking; why not take a pain pill? Ten weeks out, and routine pain medication is not in my recovery plan. It is a personal decision when narcotics for pain management is involved. I had previously experienced withdrawal symptoms after an invasive surgery with only four days of medication usage. I am too tired to have to deal with the issue of withdrawals, at the end of all this. So I will pass on narcotics for now. The surgery provided the additional diagnostic knowledge for my physicians, myself, and my family. A peace of mind for myself and family for sure.

Mid-vacation we rented a pontoon boat and picnicked in the middle of the lake. The grandkids had huge smiles as they took turns driving the boat while sitting on grandpa's lap. Once lunch was finished, of course sunscreen applied to all, a quick swim was underway. So life vests and float tubes were on, the jumping and splashing began, as one by one the grown kids cannon-balled their way into the water. One by one the grandkids either jumped in or were lowered in, but all of them wanted to play. I was so excited to take part and join the entire family (except for grandpa idling close) in the lake. Until I suddenly realized I may be able to ever so gently get into the water but would not be able to climb back as there was no ladder. So as it stood, the husbands were going to have to double-team to get everyone out of the water and back onto the boat one by one. Needing to pull on both of the arms to do so.

The frolicking continued while I was only a mere observer. Then one by one, as everyone was plucked out of the water and back on the boat, I felt one tear stream down my cheek. By the way—I know, I know I am thankful to be alive, but you never know when these incidental moments are going to happen—the tear just happens. Something touches you and before you even realize it, the tear has already made its way down the cheek. I know this sounds so ridiculous. My youngest daughter must have noticed me wipe away a tear under my sunglasses, so she said, "It's going to be all right, Mom. Don't be sad." How intuitive she was knowing how I felt missing out on something I really love to do. Although it would most likely only be a temporary limitation, it was one of those firsts, I realized I could not do. With my tears brushed away, I looked around at the smiles and laughter in the boat. My little family whom I cherish and love so much are all here with me. Then there was the captivating scenery that included a crystal blue sky, evergreen trees surrounding us with jutted peaks of exposed granite, and the breath of fresh mountain air. I paused and thanked God for this very moment.

Again I reminded myself to thank Him first about everything good in my life and complain later. This is a great habit to be in: you find you com-plain less, and it really does work. But for the purpose of this book I am sharing my thoughts, my frustrations and complaints that have been real. I'm trying to implement this new habit, and a change of habits take time. Then I recited again, 'Before I bring my needs I will bring my praise, and I will remember to thank Him for all that is good in my life.' And once I did that, it felt like He just gave me a perfect day.

Spiritual Pearl ~ Eight

Can we always recognize and appreciate even the smallest gifts we have in our lives? The little fleeting special moments should not be taken for granted. Simple things in life too, like a smile or a giggle. I just love giggles—they are so genuine—even if the smile isn't your own. It is not that hard to put a smile on. So I think about all my little favorite things in life and there are so many, so I smile. If we are thankful for each moment and in our trials, and praise Him for what He is going to do, we will be heard. Then this faithfulness will open the door to His audience. Being near Him in this way, knowing He has 'got this,' will bring us blessings of abundant joy. Then peace will be experienced and flow from this intimate welcome. Can we even imagine when He sees the joy within our hearts, what His own heart must experience? If two hearts collided, there could only be an endless flow of goodness and happiness felt from deep within our souls, and then we would exude a joy surely to be recognized by all those around us.

CHAPTER SEVENTEEN

WEEK TWELVE POST-OP

THREE MONTHS POST-OP, RETURN APPOINTMENT

I was on my return visit to Stanford to follow up after my drain removal for a hematoma and I still feel quite exhausted. My limitations, discomforts in various degrees from my arm, and the many appointments had contributed to this I was sure. I felt like I have been dealing with one thing after another for some time now, beginning last September with the start of a breast infection, then pneumonia and so on. So, yes, I was still tired, I looked tired, and I felt like a broken record.

As I waited for my husband to park the car, I overheard a mother who was pushing her son in a wheelchair telling the nurse to make sure the doctor checks his port as it was bothering him. He appeared to be around ten or eleven years old, pale, frail, bald, appeared extremely fatigued, and his 'port was bothering him.' I was sure he was receiving chemotherapy or some kind of infusion therapy. All the mother could do was convey a concern. She cannot wish this away, make him well, nor carry the burden for her little boy. She was utterly powerless. A circumstance that was completely out of her control and all she could do was love on him, and I hoped—pray. Oh, how that must feel! My heart aches thinking about it. I am sure she would change places with him in a heartbeat, as many mothers and fathers would do. Why do children get cancer? I don't know, but I wish it could discriminate.

All along I felt I have kept things in perspective and have been extremely grateful for the early catch of my cancer. I don't feel I have complained too much about my ailments to those around me, but I have included my frustrations for the purpose of this book. I have not suffered the abyss of depression that a devastating illness can bring. Sometimes I don't feel I am being very strong, though, and maybe my fatigue plays a role in this. But I have seen others suffer with it, like my dear father-in-law. I recognize I am only human and not wonder woman, and this is a challenge for me both physically and mentally. When I saw this little boy and heard the concern in the voice of his mother, my heart began to ache for both of them. Well, my fatigue and pain of these past many months suddenly didn't weigh as heavily on me, as I tried to imagine what they were each going through. We cannot know what someone is going through, unless we have walked in their shoes and lived under their life circumstances. So I prayed and ended it with "God bless all the children in the world, hold them close, and keep them wrapped in your strong loving arms."

Spiritual Pearl ~ Nine

We will never be in control of our own circumstances. It is hard to give the control to someone else, let alone by blind faith. I find my absolute trust in Him came when I realized I could not change ANY outcome of what is to be. When anxious moments set in, I would rest in the Word. The outcome of such trials may not be what we are expecting or wishing for. But knowing He could heal anything if it served His purpose, He will do so. We may experience a thousand lonely days and restless nights before we finally surrender to Him and welcome His Promises. These trials in life, however long they may take, will be His mercy in disguise. Until we realize how much we need Him, and we can lay it all down before Him by completely surrendering, we will not feel His presence. He patiently waits for us to call, and He is mighty and able to carry ALL of our burdens.

So when our journey meets the trials in this life and the struggles are real and all-consuming, try whispering His name, "Jesus." His ears will hear our even faint whisper. Our trek will most certainly prove to have unsteady footing, and plodding ahead will be fatiguing. Our instincts will be to stop dead in our tracks, and pulling out of these arduous challenges will only lead to self-pity. Pity will lead to the abyss of depression, and its grip is filled with fear and darkness. All He wants is *one more step* out of us, while HE holds our hand. His reach is infinite and has no limits in distance. He can reach for us wherever we are, and will provide the strength and direction we will require. One breath at a time, one step at a time, and one day at a time. The light unto our path will lead to abundant, fearless, love-filled life; with each step this joy becomes nearer, and we are almost at the peak.

FOLLOW-UP APPOINTMENT

Four weeks after my hospitalization, I returned for a follow-up appointment. I was ready in the exam room and she entered. I was doing better, the redness was still there but dissipating. I had completed all my antibiotics, and had one physical therapy session two days prior to this visit, which did not increase the redness over my chest at all for the first time. I was sure I appeared tired, but my pain and discomfort had improved some with draining of the hematoma. She did another in-office ultrasound of the axillary area, and we all saw the hematoma was now only a third of the original size. Slowly my body was trying to reabsorb and break it all down. This was good news yet again. But the redness was still hanging around. I know she would remember this, as I asked her if I could share my thoughts on what was going on. She had never seen this reaction before either. I informed her of the sequence of events and kept in mind my activity, the research, physiological understanding I had interpreted, and shared my thoughts. I discussed with her what I concluded had contributed to my body's reaction. I was also encouraged that during all of this, there was never any presence of an infection. I never had a fever.

To me, this was all a physiological response to the presence of blood and all else mentioned above. So we entertained the possibility of getting back in the pool and continuing with weekly physical therapy. What would the risk be, if any? The goal would be to get the remainder of blood moving sooner than later. I might notice an increase in redness, but only temporarily and eventually it would have to stop. Again, there was no infection present, there was no new blood, so why not? Almost with enthusiasm I said to them, "Let's not forget the physiological possibility of all this. If we can get any of the remaining blood moved out, with exercise (swimming) or massage and by encouraging what is left to seep into the tissue, it will eventually be reabsorbed." I felt it could aid in a quicker recovery for me. They would say it made sense and let's try it. So she gave me the green light to return to swimming, as the drain site had completely healed. I had been careful with my wound care and the drain site was completely healed over. I would resume swimming.

I left the office saying, "Note to self: when you encounter another patient with this unexplained 'radiation like' rash similar to mine, and no fever or sign of infection, suspect an underlying hematoma." I truly enjoyed my visit with my surgeon and her nurse. Both have been talented, caring, and supportive for sure. There is always something we providers see for the first time even if we have done the same procedure hundreds of times. No two patients are alike. Believe me when I say we have many 'note-to-self' moments in medicine. I had antibiotics on standby, and would start them if I noted any sign of spreading occurring or beginning fever. I resumed with my swims and had physical therapy once a week. The redness in my chest, breast, and abdomen took time resolving completely. This was a slow process for the body to break this down and for reabsorption to occur. Don't get discouraged if you are experiencing the same thing. It will go away in time. It took an extra three to four weeks, maybe slightly longer, for the redness in the skin to return to normal. However, my breast lymph swelling is a completely different issue.

THE BOOK BECOMES AN IDEA

It's early August: the idea of a 'possible' book began to take shape. As I shared some of the Holy Spirit moments with family and friends, they kept saying, "You need to write about it. I wasn't quite sure how I could or if I would be able to incorporate the two topics, which became my life the entire past year. But as I experienced one Holy Spirit moment after another, His presence ever apparent with the synchronization of my spiritual walk and medical recovery, I knew it had to be possible. The question would lie on whether I am good enough as an author and this story be worth reading. I decided to just try and incorporate my scripture journaling with my chronological medical walk through my course with melanoma, and see if it started to sound worthwhile. So I began to write in August and kept fueling my heart with scripture. Through Him all things are possible! Eventually once again I felt the Holy Spirit provide direction for the book, and I was determined to finish it in the form of a twofold topic.

It twisted and turned at first, requiring tweaking multiple times, but as I sit here today just a couple weeks away from trying to find publishing, I am proud of it. It was a great experience to write and see all the Holy Spirit moments throughout the journey empowering me in more ways than one. Sometimes we amaze ourselves too: where is this coming from? But I know the answer. I would ask my husband and say, "Will you listen to what I just wrote and tell me what you think?" He of course always said yes. He was always encouraging and proud of me. He would listen and give me feedback, but he genuinely seemed to like what I was writing. He reads a lot, and the chapters that I shared with him he thought became more gripping. Those were his words, and maybe he couldn't hurt my feelings. He offered suggestions so I kept praying and writing, and suddenly I was almost finished with it. Once I have my 'missile lock' on, I will see it through to the end. Another part of my personality: perseverance and relentlessness. If you're reading it, then it has been published and I hope you've learned just one thing. The 'one thing' is your call.

TWO INTERESTING QUESTIONS - UNIVERSAL PHENOMENA

There have been many reasons for my desire to discover new things, especially spiritual reasons, during this challenge, as my focus on Him gave me encouragement through the months and has made me stronger. He promises to be near, and He is nearer than I realize. But during this journey, I also find myself fascinated by the mechanics of our body and the complex functionality and intertwined systems within it. I am in continued awe of His work, because I believe it is His work.

The interactions and dialogues I have had with so many knowledgeable physicians explaining the 'who, what, when, where, how, and why' to me makes it obvious to me that my little brain and its IQ is no match. I am thankful for the brilliant scientists and geneticists who have dedicated and contributed their efforts in this arena of medicine. I have grasped the basic understanding of the anatomy and physiology of my diagnosis and what I am going through. I conclude, even with the addition of all this new knowledge, I still prefer being the provider as opposed to being the patient.

But while I am in awe of the expertise I have encountered, I find I am ... there isn't even a word to really capture nor describe the magnitude of the achievement He has bestowed upon this universe, including creating these brilliant minds. But especially when it comes to creating each of us, in His image. Creation of the human being. The complexities of each system, down to the genetic mapping of our DNA, will forever remain beyond my comprehension. I have taken the beauty of how my body performs for granted, good or bad. Even with all my past education—from obstetrics (I have always been in awe of following the growth of a fetus in utero via ultrasound, and the miracle of birth), gynecology, reproductive endocrinology, to basic dermatology—there is always more to learn. I know I will never completely understand it all, but I will forever be intrigued by His perfect design.

This is one reason why I found the book by Dr. Francis S. Collins, *The Language of God*, so fascinating. The project was to unveil the complete genetic mapping of the human being. The author is also a brilliant geneticist and the lead in the Human Genome Project. He is struck with the realization that God was the only one with the original blue print. His personal and scientific discoveries during his role as the lead geneticists provide a thought-provoking and engaging read, as he felt so humbled to have successfully accomplished this with his team. As he journeyed through ten years on the project, he had a spiritual awakening of his own. As he began questioning the possible existence of God, journaling and wanting the results to be a factual discovery, he was certain he would find substantial proof to refute this. During this time he was encouraged to read a book, *Mere Christianity*, by C.S. Lewis. In reading C.S. Lewis's writings, he was intrigued as he reflected on a couple of questions. Questions that could not be answered, but would lie open-ended for you to decide what the answer SHOULD be. This led him on a path he was not expecting either, a spiritual one. In the end found himself in awe of our Creator.

The first question was actually scientifically researched from all corners of the world: how is it that *universally*, people know right from wrong? The moral law.

This first question on knowing the difference between right and wrong does not mean people always do what is right. Hence the bad or evil in the world. But I do believe we are born with an inherent instinct to know the difference between a right and a wrong. I feel it. You probably feel it also. What makes people respond to the same situation differently? Is it life circumstances, environments, other challenges contributing to and influencing our choices? But sometimes a wrong is equal to a sin in God's eyes.

Reading *The Language of God*, I find Dr. Collins elaborates on the concept of right versus wrong even more. I have never thought about it before and it has become quite thought-provoking. I do wonder *what type of influence* is behind our desire (most of us) to do what is right. C.S. Lewis, in his book *Mere Christianity* addresses the moral law. The real question lies with: why? Why is this innate and built into our persona in the first place? What is it for those of us who are conscientiously aware or concerned of always doing what is right? If we are not faith-based believers, then who are we appealing to? There is a higher standard here and a universal phenomenon to abide by it. And could there be an influencing 'force' behind it? This is called the moral law, or the law of right behavior: does this have an unmeasurable value, where there is no scientific tool to measure it if in fact this is an intrinsic, invisible, faith-driven character trait introduced within us and supported only by a higher power? The concept of right and wrong appears to be universal among all members of the human species. Universal, among all members of humanity. Now obviously there are people who make choices to do wrong and evil things. So, did they not inherit this invisible gene, the law of right behavior, or were there outside influencing forces and factors that drove them to an alternate decision in choices of behavior?

It became clear to Collins that if God exists, then He must be outside the natural world, and therefore the tools of science are not adequate tools to learn about Him. The moral law argument forced him to admit the plausibility of the God Hypothesis. Dr. Collins concluded that faith in God seemed more rational than an agnostic view. He accepted the possibility of a spiritual world view to include the existence of God.

Spiritual Pearl ~ Ten

My spiritual thoughts on this first question goes way back to a story many of us have already heard. We probably haven't given it a second thought, but could this Good vs. Evil (right versus wrong) theme stem from the Garden of Eden? This according to scripture was in the beginning when God made man and then woman from man's rib. They both were aware of God's command. Now introduce a third party, the serpent, who persuades Eve that surely God would not mean for her to die if she eats from this tree. So the story continues.

> *And the Lord God commanded the man, "You are free to eat from any tree in the garden; but you must not eat from the tree of the knowledge of good and evil, for when you eat from it you will certainly die,"*
> GEN 2:16–17

The woman said to the serpent, "We may eat fruit from the trees in the garden, but God did say, 'You must not eat fruit from the tree that is in the middle of the garden, and you must not touch it, or you will die,'"

GEN 3:2-3

We know how the story goes: when questioned by God in the Garden of Eden, Adam and Eve are hiding, as they are ashamed, embarrassed at being naked. Eve tells God she was deceived by the serpent to eat the apple fruit from the tree of knowledge of good and evil. Adam tells God that Eve made him do it. He says;

"The woman you put here with me-she gave me some fruit from the tree, and I ate it,"

GEN 3:12

I can elaborate in so many different directions here, which actually may be really funny. But Adam takes no responsibility for his own actions. Temptation is introduced. Eve disobeyed, shame and embarrassment immediately set in, and our Lord set the consequence for both of their disobedience. At that moment God knew, as He gave the gift of choice to Adam and Eve, and in doing so He also knew we would inevitably sin. We will all do a 'wrong' at some time in our life. Some wrongs are just more damaging than others. The temptations of this world are great, easily accessible, and will always be there. He needed to deliver all of us from sins of all past, present, and future with the ransom of His Son, Jesus Christ, by the shedding of His blood on the cross, for all mankind, in order for us to be with Him in Heaven for Eternity.

So do we think we will be held to a higher standard? Or do we know we will be held to a higher standard? Those are two very different questions. Being unsure is okay. But just don't let it stop there. Spend the time to find out. If God cannot be measured by any scientific tools, does that mean He does not exist or just that He is not of this world?

"Without faith it is impossible to please God, because anyone who comes to him must believe that he exists and that he rewards those who earnestly seek him,"

HEB 11:6

Just give God a glance and that is all you need to make the right choice. WWJD. What would Jesus do?

The second question pondered by Dr. Collins also scientifically researched but again with no scientific tool to measure this by is: why do we universally have this natural instinct to love? We can feel love. We want to love. We can give love. We enjoy receiving love by others. We want to be loved. But why? Why is this within most of us? My spiritual thought here is contained in one sentence: because HE FIRST LOVED US. That is it, and it is powerful.

"We love because he first loved us."

1 JOHN 4:19, NIV

Let yourself meditate on this for a moment.

CHAPTER EIGHTEEN

FOUR TO SIX MONTHS POST-OP

FOUR MONTHS POST-OP

How easy it is to slip back into an old habit. Of course it is in the moments I am distracted and all consumed with self that old habits creep back into my mind. This is a reminder of how humanly flawed I am. But as my arm did not provide me relief and freedom from pain, I got so discouraged. Again this month was better than last month. But seriously I was hoping for more relief by this time.

I can really appreciate the fluctuations in my emotional lability during this new health challenge. When I am thankful and focused on His Promises to me, it is hope that penetrates my mind. But when I am distracted by the solitude and confinement of my recovery setbacks, I have a wondering mind and self-pity moments. I have had many friends who assure me a pity party is a normal occurrence: it is a human response. I get that, but having a pity party is new to me. I can't remember when I thought I had one last. However, the medical person in me thinks at times if this 'party' doesn't last long (what is too long?) and one can control the depths this self-pity can take you, it can be healthy for a recovery. You know, like sometimes a good cry is all you need. After all, the current trial and struggle is real, and coping with all the changes is a very gradual process, requiring patience. Everyone grieves the loss of what was once considered normal to them at some point, until the new normal can become clear. This takes time (see, I just said it again to myself): a patient needs patience and practice in adjusting to new ways of doing things or accepting the permanent challenge, with tolerance of the pain and discomfort a part of it.

This is the same time frame when my husband and I were preparing to put my mother-in-law's home on the market. Within two weeks of my drain being removed, he and I cleaned out her entire home (me with one arm), donated what needed to be donated, and came across memories of a life well lived. This home was filled with love and treasures. The large family photo with over thirty-two of us in the picture was taken on a vacation, hung over her fireplace. I was sad she was gone, but I was very thankful she did not suffer as my father-in-law had. The past holds dear memories that we will not forget. Isn't that also a wonderful gift, to be able to recall the good memories in life? I find myself melancholic off and on as we prepare for her 'Celebration of Life' service in a couple of weeks.

While I myself did not experience depression with my challenge, I know others can with theirs. The medical provider in me is why I wish to include this. It can be a struggle for some and an extremely difficult struggle for others. Other than the constant discomfort in the arm and incision area, I was doing quite well. It was my impatience once again with how slowly I felt I was recovering that continues to agitate me. Again, I must continue to remind myself, I have had a major insult to my arm. I just need more time.

The grieving process is clear, and is not experienced ONLY with the loss of a loved one. It can be experienced with any major stressor in life: a move, loss of a job or home, etc., financial struggle, sudden health issue, a tragic accident, and more. All are circumstances that require one to adjust to a major change. These basic and identified five stages—denial, anger, bargaining, depression, and acceptance—are all a part of the natural process of adjusting to a loss or crisis of some kind. They help identify the way we are feeling, and there is no timeline to work through these stages and toward the reality of a new normal. Everyone's timeline will be different, the circumstance for the grief will differ, and with that, somedays are better than others. So setbacks for some can be expected. Struggling with any type of grief, especially alone I would assume, is extremely difficult.

Physicians will say, and I did as well, there is no timeline to grieve. But it is the timeline that can become a critical factor. If the sadness becomes wallowing and is not waning and other symptoms begin to appear and take hold, then there may be an issue ensuing. That is what makes all the difference in a healthy recovery of the heart and especially the mind. There is a fine line between normal grieving associated with a stressor, in this case loss of a loved one and cancer, versus the onset of a chronic mental health issue. Sometimes the devastation of the illness can trigger depression to set in, and most people are unprepared with how to emotionally cope during the trek through all the tough days that lie ahead. Your fuel is emptying, the car is riding on fumes. This is when emotional turmoil comes to visit. How long the visit lasts, depends. Depends on coping skills.

We as providers try and stay attuned to this with patients. Almost all my physicians at Stanford asked how I was adjusting mentally to my newfound health situation. They made me take a five- to seven-question, questionnaire to see if I showed signs of depression. They suggested yoga, meditation, or engaging in a new hobby. All great suggestions for distracting and relaxing the mind. I have chosen to embark on a spiritual journey. You may want to consider one of these or all of these avenues to help in coping with the 'new' normal in your life. How to refuel as mentioned before is really necessary and may be a vital factor.

When situational depression turns into a chronic depression, it can be a very dark place that requires professional intervention. My prayer is for **any of you reading this right now who feel you just can't seem to cope with your struggle to make an appointment with your doctor.** Be specific with your complaint when you go in for your appointment. All you need to say is, 'I feel sad all the time.' If they don't seem to help you, then ask for a referral or find another doctor. Sometimes I don't understand the fear or trepidation some physicians have in treating depression. I have witnessed the benefits of this over and over in both private practice and at the college campus level. The intervention with medication may be temporary: it doesn't mean you have to be on medication forever. But finding a physician who understands the different medications and can educate you on the treatment plan, side effects, and warning signs is important, and may be challenging. If they don't feel comfortable in this area, then ask them to refer you to someone who can help and hang in there during this process. Counseling is a necessary part of the plan whenever medication is involved. Whether it is back with the provider who started you on medication or referral to a psychologist, it is key in monitoring.

How I would cope if my news was more devastating, like maybe some of you reading this, I don't know. But I do know this: I have someone to lean on and take that burden from me. I have surrendered. I will count on Him and seek Him out should the time come. One day it will. So until that time comes, I need to maintain a good routine with my visits with Him. I am usually a very positive person, outgoing, very comfortable with who I am and what defines me. But even the strongest of mind with faith in hand can have moments of feeling overwhelmed, frustrated, and lonely. I am impatient with my limitations, and I cannot do what I used to be able to do. This last setback with the hematoma, hospitalization, and loss of blood was so discouraging, confining, and exhausting. I do not like feeling like a caged bird. My husband would say a "caged lioness," not a caged bird.

SIX MONTHS POST-OP

Surveillance Recommendations and Lymphedema

There are many surveillance avenues for monitoring skin changes. These are but a couple which can prove to be helpful to say the least. Even I discovered the smallest of small melanoma lesion with a routine skin self-exam. Just as you should be in a routine for doing your monthly breast exam, you need to get in the habit of doing a skin self-exam as well. Get to know your skin and its little kisses from God!

Mole Mapping: This is a painless and noninvasive tool to help track changes in moles and detect melanoma. This digital photoimaging tool can aid in early intervention as changes can be identified. It is a surveillance program usually offered by a dermatologist to persons with a moderate to excessive amount of freckles as well as those who are high-risk for melanoma. I don't know if this is considered a covered benefit on insurance plans.

Skin self-exams: Once a full body exam is done by a dermatologist, they can ins truct you how to do a thorough skin self-exam. You do this in the comfort of your own home, with hand mirror and full length mirror, bright light, pencil, ruler, blow dryer, a chair to sit in as you inspect your legs, body maps that your dermatologist can give you.

- Do this at minimum every 6–8 weeks, to get to know your body patterns, marks, freckles, sores, lumps or changes in your skin, flakiness, sores that bleed off and on
- Examine your face, pay attention to your nose, lips, ears both front and back
- With your comb and blow dryer inspect your scalp. You may ask your hairdresser if she or he notices any freckles or unusual lesions on your head when they style your hair
- Look at your hands—between the fingers and toes, under your fingernails, then move up the front and back of your arms
- In front of a full-length mirror, begin at the elbows and raise your arms up, checking both front and back of the arm and underarms
- Focus on the neck, chest, and torso. Women don't forget to look under the breasts as well, so lift them
- With your handheld mirror, check out your back in the full-length mirror and inspect the neck first working your way down shoulders, upper back, upper back of the arms and sides
- Still using the mirrors check your lower back out, buttock, and back of the legs
- Sitting down, examine the front and back of the legs, between your legs, then move down to thigh and down to your toes. Inspect both front and back. Check between your toes and inspect your nailbeds

- Get a body map from your dermatologist and map this out as instructed; you will need a ruler to try and measure the size of lesions (moles, freckles, sores)

Then there are more diagnostic tests for surveillance monitoring of the cancer that are typically ordered by your managing physician. These include the PET scan, brain MRIs, and L-Dex tests.

Surveillance Continues with PET scans, MRIs, and L-Dex Testing

The second of three rounds of brain scans and PET scans both returned negative. Another blessing. My overall condition was stable, with the ongoing arm discomfort from either webbing as we discussed earlier or some nerve pain that came and went. The L-Dex testing showed the swelling in my arm was creeping its way up a little. When these numbers change, it might be the first sign that swelling was around the corner. Hence, why they follow these reading three times in the first year for comparison and measure it to the baseline obtained prior to the surgery. You should have had the same testing done. Which meant I must wear my sleeve a little more than I was used to.

What is Lymphedema? It is an abnormal buildup of fluid and cell wastes in the tissue that occurs when the lymph system is unable to function properly for many different reasons. This will usually occur in the extremity that has been compromised. In my case, surgery to the left axillary region would interrupt the flow in my left arm.

There are various stages of lymphedema which I am not going to get into as your physician is better qualified to inform you of your risks and stage with you. The risk of developing lymphedema postoperatively varies from patient to patient and it is difficult to say who will most likely experience this swelling during their recovery. Some patients will experience irreversible effects of the condition for many reasons and others will not.

Individual anatomical differences, extent of surgery, infection, trauma and treatments like radiation influence the structural and functional capabilities of the lymphatic system which play a role in the risk with this condition. Lymphedema may not present as a complication right away, but can appear within a few months to a few years. **Following the postoperative instructions given to you by your physician and paying attention to the signs and symptoms of lymphedema after surgery, will be important.**

This is why the L-Dex test is done prior the surgery and every three months after the surgery, to gauge if this is beginning to become an issue.

I have experienced the early stages of lymphedema with some firmness and swelling to varying degrees. There is always associated pain and fullness in my upper arm. My elbow will ache from time to time, various sensations are felt and the breast tissue was the escape route for the overflow of fluid. The rerouting of fluid may take many weeks if not months to occur. My diligence in following postop instructions, wearing my sleeve when I noticed these changes, along with lymphatic physical therapy may have played a role in readily reversing those ontoward symptoms. Paying attention to the symptomatology in my arm is a daily routine. Remember this will be a part of your body that may have difficulty fighting off infections like it used to, so you have to be extra careful and rethink how you might do things. Be protective of this limb or area. Helpful hints regarding lymphedema will be shared towards the end of this chapter.

Lymphedema Specialist: I have a new kind of appointment awaiting me at Stanford in February of 2018: I will meet a physician who specializes in lymphedema. So I have no news for you as yet regarding what he will tell me to do that is different from what I am already doing. I will share as end points in the next chapter. I am curious though, and my first questions will be: If I am on blood pressure medication which at times causes a little dependent swelling of my ankles, especially if I am sitting for a few hours (like in a car ride), how does this L-Dex test know the difference in the cellular swelling?

The following guides I have accumulated from different resources which I found helpful. Many tips and warnings can be found online. I read so many different ones and started to jot down notes. **Nothing should ever replace the specific instructions your physician has reviewed with you.** In reading these, they must become second nature when the lymph system has suffered such an insult.

Lymphedema

It should always be first and foremost on our mind to take the best care possible of our extremity that is compromised.

Signs/Symptoms of Lymphedema of the ARM (Your physician should have a handout for you regarding the symptoms they would want to be notified about. ALWAYS FOLLOW their advice as they are familiar with your specific needs and your health issue)

- Begins with a sensory change like tingling or numbing in the arm for one or two days then goes away and recurs again
- You notice your rings are getting tight or don't fit anymore
- Achiness, tingling, discomfort, increase warmth on the hand, chest, or underarm
- Feeling of fullness in any part of the arm
- Tightness or decreased flexibility in any joint area
- Bursting or shooting pains, pins and needles
- Tenderness in the elbow region
- Slight puffiness or swelling in the arm, hand or chest - pitting edema
- Veins are harder to see, knuckles also, skin appears smoother
- Clothing, especially sleeve is tighter, bra feels tighter and leaves indentations
- The back area looks asymmetrical
- Can't slip jewelry off and on as usual
- Changes in skin texture and appearance, tight, red hardening
- Rash, itching, redness, pain and warmth
- Fever and flulike symptoms

NOTIFY YOUR PHYSICIAN IMMEDIATELY FOR EVALUATION IF ANY OF THE ABOVE ARE EXPERIENCED

Lymphedema Suggestions and Precautions

Your physician should have a handout for you regarding these suggestions and precautions, and ALWAYS FOLLOW their advice for they are familiar with your specific needs and your health issue.

- Good hygiene. Keeping the skin healthy, clean (Dove is a good soap that is slightly acidic and better for your skin, but you can ask your physician what they prefer you use) and dry thoroughly. Properly hydrate the skin with lotion EVERY DAY using a low pH lotion like: Eucerin, Curel, Dermal therapy, Lac-Hydrin, or Johnson & Johnson baby lotion
- Check your skin frequently and make sure there is no new cuts, open wounds, bites, redness or infections noted. If you notice a cut, wash with soap and water, apply antiseptic ointment and cover with Band-Aid. If there is no improvement and signs of infection, contact your physician
- For any new changes in the extremity, swelling, cracking especially in the creases or areas of numbness, contact your physician
- Keep your nailbeds and cuticles in good condition and watch for infection. Do not cut, pick or tear at your cuticles. If you are wearing artificial nails, make sure your salon is using disinfected instruments
- Consider using and over-the-counter antifungal for the feet in cases with lymphedema of the leg
- Wear clean clothing, always. Compression garments should be worn once and washed every day
- Wear extra-long oven mitts when cooking. Be careful of steam burns when opening the microwave, and use CLEAN gloves when washing dishes, loading the dishwasher, doing household cleaning

chores, using chemical cleansers (this can be harsh on the skin and cause it to crack), outdoor yardwork, or gardening

- Shave using an electric razor if possible, for armpits, legs, and bikini area. Razors can cause nicks and cuts. Use disposable razors each time and start with area at risk first—this will minimize risk of infection with a clean blade. However, if lymphedema is really bad, recommend avoidance altogether
- Use a thimble if sewing or mending
- Use insect repellant in areas where bites are more likely
- Swim ONLY in a clean pool, and do not swim if you have open sores on the effected arm
- Use your effected limb as normally as possible
- Exercise moderately in the morning or afternoon and avoid the heat of midday, but begin slowly and increasing gradually while monitoring any changes in your limb, size, shape, tissue, texture, soreness, heaviness, or firmness. Wear compression garments for strenuous activity, running, prolonged standing, weight lifting
- Maintain an optimal weight
- Use SPF as discussed earlier and as directed by your physician. Even on cloudy days, apply your sunscreen
- Make sure to avoid scalding burns and watch the water temperature in your own home
- Wear loose jewelry and watches, but preferably wear them on the opposite arm. Do not wear any jewelry to bed for precautionary measure
- Carry your purse, grocery bags, and grandchildren on the OPPOSITE arm. Lighten the load when you can in your purse. Avoid tugging or pulling heavy loads
- Wear a properly measured compression garment when flying, and drink plenty of water, minimize your sodium intake, walk about the cabin when it is safely permitted, anything to help to decrease swelling
- Hot tubs, Jacuzzi, steam baths and saunas may not be used. Personal Jacuzzis may be used with moderate temperature

- Wear loose clothing and not clothing that will be constricting to other areas of your body. Avoid tight elastic bra straps. They must not dig into the shoulders. Anything that acts like a tourniquet will increase swelling
- NEVER allow blood pressure to be taken on the effected arm, NOR blood punctures for blood draws
- Discuss what type of diet your health care provider prefers you to be on and follow their instructions. Healthy balance diets are available on the American Heart Association or American Cancer Association web sites for guidelines. Otherwise, a low fat, low sodium, and high-fiber diet is suggested. Avoid tobacco, alcohol, and caffeine, drink adequate water
- CALL YOUR PHYSICIAN **IMMEDIATELY** IF YOU HAVE THE FOLLOWING:
- Redness at a site you don't usually have, part or all of your arm or leg is warmer or hotter than usual
- You have new or different pain in your arm or leg, or have red streaking
- You have more swelling than usual
- Fever or flulike symptoms or you feel unwell

Self-massage of Remaining Lymph Regions/ Basins/Depots

This will assist with lymph circulation and should be done prior to exercise and throughout the day. Massage slowly and softly, gently moving the skin and NOT pressing down hard over the area.

1. **Sternoclavicular Fossa** - this is the area right above your clavicle (collarbone). With fingers flat, circle above the collar bone, softly moving your hand in a circular motion from the outside of the clavicle toward your neck. Repeat this 10 times and do the opposite side.
2. **Axilla** - the remaining armpit area. With your hand flat under

the armpit, gently circle toward your trunk, moving only the skin. Release and repeat 10 times

3. **Abdomen** - place your hands on the center of your stomach, right at the belly button. As you take a breath in, allow your stomach to rise as you inhale with air. Let your hands rise with it, then as you exhale, gently press down and release. Repeat this 10 times

4. **Inguinal,** place both hands on each side of your groin. Stroke gently upward toward your belly button. This stroke should be firmer than all the previous areas you have massaged. Repeat this 10 times

UPDATES FOR AUGUST

Many appointments consumed my next several weeks as my condition remained slowly improving. I never saw improvement day to day, but more like month to month. So remember that recovering is a tedious waiting period. This month feels better than the last. So try and be patient, and I know that is easier said than done. Then I had a setback of shingles in September, which ran its routine course. I will explain these signs and symptoms also. Immuno-compromised system, stress from the whole ordeal was probably the leading cause why I came down with shingles. I know, right—no fun.

Cutaneous Oncology Surgeon: I have had a follow-up appointment with my surgeon who specializes in lymph node dissections and other surgeries. She is happy with my resolve of the hematoma and wound healing. The incision site under the arm is well healed and fading. The incisions on my back are well healed and barely noticeable even though both were four-and-a-half-inch scars. What an amazing skill she has, with precision and technique. I was ever so thankful she came recommended to me. I was released from her care and she referred me for continued physical therapy. I do recommend physical therapy to be started as soon as possible once post-op recovery appears stable. I began around the five-week mark. The technique of a certified lymphatic massage therapist is helpful. Rubbing/stroking your arm with one hand is not as effective, but most times it is all we can do. So do this daily.

Specialist Breast Surgeon: my appointment with my Stanford breast cancer specialist was encouraging. While she had never seen the exaggerated response my breast had with the filling of lymphatic fluid, she was diligent in making sure that within my PET scan, no breast cancer was present. She went the extra step and obtained my 3D breast images from my local radiologist for comparison and had them reviewed by a Stanford radiologist. My overall swelling in the breast had slowly improved, and the skin color was not as red. The yellowish hue was a little less than before. This breast recovery had been the slowest of slow processes as I mention over and over. As for the abscess, she was following this as well. There had been improvement. I would be following up with her nurse practitioner in late November for a quick check. They want to use this as a learning moment and experience my progress for future 'note to self' moments. Witnessing the post-op course with me and the recovery it took to finally resolve is always educational. We may choose to use this for the purpose of encouragement to subsequent patients who may go through the same thing. Anytime you find a physician who will take a second look at something just to be sure it is not of deeper concern, keep them!

Local Breast Surgeon: my local breast surgeon has much experience in the area of breast cancer and has earned a much-deserved reputation in town. Women come from everywhere to get on her schedule. She is one of the best in town and that makes her one of the busiest around. Even my Stanford breast specialist had heard of her and had very positive things to share with me. She reviewed my 3D mammogram and repeat sonogram of the breast and both were almost back to normal. She did a thorough breast exam on me, followed by an in-office sonogram, and picked up two cysts in my right breast that I thought I had. So we would follow these over the course of several months, and I would see her back should I notice a change. Some lymph swelling in my breast continued; she had seen this before, but not to the extent of mine. Even this had improved greatly. I will continue to see her every six months. It is amazing how long an abscess can take to resolve, as the circulation in the breast is different by design. But any infectious resolve may be additionally compromised if any prior surgeries have been done to the areas, which include, but not limited to, breast implants, breast lifts or reductions, and any breast reconstruction surgeries. It has almost been one year for this abscess.

Local Oncologist: He has me checked in with him every three to six months, as I was not doing any infusion/immunotherapy treatments. He always reviewed my latest tests in more detail. He reviewed my recent PET scan and brain MRI, both of which returned negative. That made me six months clear. The next set of these would be done in late November. I would recommend having a local oncologists established, especially if you are traveling to another medical center for treatments. While I would not change a thing regarding my many appointments, team of physicians or surgical interventions at Stanford, it was a three-to-four-hour drive for me every time. And that was on a good day with traffic! I would also recommend in this age of electronic medical records to sign up with a local physician who can share and has access to the same information as your away group of physicians. There was no need for record release of information needed in this case.

Health Considerations

Other health considerations when immune-compromised all warrant discussion with your physician first.

Annual Health Exams/Vaccinations: It is important that even in the midst of all the endless appointments, we do not forget to obtain our ANNUAL routine exams and vaccinations. Vaccinations are based on age fifty and over only. **Discussion is warranted with your physician regarding all vaccinations, as there may be contraindications for receiving the injections based on your personal health history.**

Td (tetanus, diphtheria) and Tdap (tetanus, diphtheria, and pertussis) vaccine: Everyone should have the Tdap at least once, even if you are over age sixty-five and have never had it. CDC recommends a Td rebooster every ten years. There has been a rise in whooping cough, and anyone around infant younger than twelve months should be vaccinated. This includes parents, grandparents, and childcare providers. So have the discussion with your doctor. Some physicians keep up with these recommendations more than others, and if this has not been discussed with you, you need to bring it up. There may be a reason your doctor has not offered it to you in regards to personal health history.

MMR (measles, mumps, rubella) vaccine: CDC recommends this for all adults born after 1956 who have never been immunized or are unsure if they have been immunized. Also, persons born before 1957 (the year the first measles vaccine was tested) should be immune as most likely you had one of the diseases as a child. If you don't know your immunization status, get the booster shot. You only need get this ONCE. Again, consult your physician regarding this, as there may be a contraindication based on your personal health history.

Hepatitis A vaccine: CDC recommends consideration of this vaccine ONCE but given in two doses over six to eighteen months. If you have high-risk behaviors, this warrants a discussion with your physician, as there may be contraindications for receiving the vaccine based on your personal health history.

Hepatitis B vaccine: CDC recommends consideration of this vaccine ONCE but in three doses. Second injection is given 4 weeks after the first, and the third injection is given 5 months after the second. Get a booster if you are unsure of your status. This should be considered if you have a high-risk behavior and warrants further discussion with your physician as there may be contraindications for receiving the vaccination based on your personal health history. It's also recommended for persons who have jobs that expose them to blood or bodily fluids.

Meningococcal vaccine: CDC recommends consideration for all persons over the age of fifty who have never been vaccinated. If you are between fifty to fifty-five years old, then the meningococcal conjugate vaccination (MCV4) that remains effective for life. If over the age of fifty-five, then poly-saccharide vaccine (MPSV4) that provides three to five years immunity is recommended. This is administered ONCE, in one injection. Again, persons who have jobs that expose them to the disease should consider the vaccine. Discussion with your doctor is necessary as there may be contrain-dications in regards to your personal health history.

Influenza or Flu vaccination. The CDC (Center for Disease Control) rec-ommends all persons nine months of age or older get vaccinated, including pregnant women. It is important at minimum to have a discussion with your doctor whether or not you should receive it. Lymphadenectomy sur-gery (removal of one or more groups of lymph nodes) compromises the immune system. Anytime the lymph nodes are removed, the immune sys-tem will never function at its optimum capacity. Hence, we must do what we can to help our system out. If you read the vaccination is less effective than expected, it would be something to ask your physician about. Weighing the risk of getting sick vs the potential benefit of the vaccination warrants further discussion between you and the physician if there are no contrain-dications based on your personal health history.

Pneumococcal (polysaccharide) vaccine as recommended by the CDC is for adults over the age of sixty-five years and older. Persons two to sixty-four years old who are at increased risk for disease due to medical conditions, and adults nineteen through sixty-four years of age who smoke. If there are no contraindications based on your personal health history.

Zostavax/Shingles vaccine: as recommended by the CDC, all persons over the age of sixty are to receive the vaccination, as the risk for getting shingles (herpes zoster, which is the same virus that causes chickenpox, varicella zoster) and post-herpetic neuralgia (PHN) increases as we age. However, in March of 2011, the FDA ruled persons over the age of fifty (as it had already been approved for persons over the age of sixty) may receive the vaccine. According to the CDC, one out of every three persons in the United States will develop shingles in their lifetime. If there are no contraindications based on your personal health history.

Shingles—In Brief

What is **shingles?** When the chickenpox virus reactivates in the body and causes a sequential array of symptoms. It may occur in one in three adults over the age of fifty. Early symptoms include: headache, sensitivity to light, and flulike symptoms without fever. Acute pain, tingling numbness, and itching on a specific part of the skin on one side of the body will occur. You may have a band, strip, or small area with a rash or blisterlike formations that appear several days or weeks later.

This September I saw my general physician, as I was sure I was beginning a bout with shingles. This was not a fun condition. I experienced all the symptoms in the exact order of onset. The 'pain', usually unilateral (one sided)could be scalp pain, ear pain, and neck pain for the areas in the head. This is a case when the sooner symptoms can be recognized, the sooner a course of -anti-viral medications can be started. It is important NOT to ignore any of the symptoms. It ran its course for three weeks' duration, but mine was not as bad as some. Knowing my immune system had already been impacted, I recognized the symptoms immediately and started on antiviral medication. So from personal experience, I would encourage anyone with immuno-compromise over the age of fifty to contact your physician and at a minimum have a discussion about getting the vaccination. Remember, our immune system has suffered a major insult and it will make us more susceptible to anything. Including, if you remember, 'increased risk of additional skin cancers.' Otherwise, the vaccination should be considered at the age of sixty. The injection will not protect us 100 percent against getting shingles, but it will aid in decreasing the risk in a reactivation of the virus within our system.

My Advice: Common Sense Approach

This advice is to help reduce the risk of lymphedema, not prevent it. Risk reduction should always be individualized. Always follow the advice of your physician.

Physical Therapy: I would recommend starting this as soon as you have had some initial recovery time. Maybe by 5 or 6 weeks postoperative. Sooner if you feel pretty well, but it will be between you and your physician. I have continued with my physical therapy and exercise. When engaging in physical therapy, making sure your therapist is a certified lymphedema therapist (CLT) is important. They understand the lymphatic system and its circulation. They understand the importance of the gentle or 'stroking' method to massage with movement of the skin and not the muscle. We should not have an aggressive massage to the injured arm, as this may actually damage the remaining lymph nodes. Lymph nodes are very delicate and we need all the remaining nodes to function like they are supposed to. I try and do the lymph massage as I described earlier, to the remaining lymph node sites, to aid in activating the nodes and promoting rerouting of lymph fluid when I remember.

Exercise: Swimming is very therapeutic and would have to be my number one recommendation for therapy of the upper arm. It is a sport that provides a natural compression element on the arm during a workout where gravity pull has less of an impact. You don't have to be a fast swimmer to get the benefit of this exercise. Simply being in the pool and doing some breaststroke is enough, or floating on your back and letting your arms float above your head then slowly pulling downward, like making a snow angle in the water. I really notice a difference in flexibility and improved comfort when lifting my arms. If I don't continue to do my exercises, I can notice the increase discomfort in my arm. I have tried to swim at least two to three times a week. If I don't overdo it with the amount of yardage I swim, my arm feels so much better. Baby steps with my swimming and I gradually built up to a more challenging workout. But my swimming routine doesn't always work out, with reasons beyond my control; winter months are difficult for at times the weather is miserable to swim in an outdoor pool. So summer months will be easier, even increasing this amount per week will be helpful. If the pool appears too dirty, as the pump is malfunctioning, I will absolutely avoid this exposure, or the heater may be out. I also swim with a long-sleeved swim shirt on and wear sunscreen on my exposed skin areas, face, and legs. I will swim before 10:00 AM also. I like being outdoors and I love to swim, and some of my best ideas come to me in the stillness under the water. So this is my compromise.

Walking: If swimming is not possible, then a good walk is great. I try not to swing my injured arm while walking. But keeping your legs strong is great also and considered a weight-bearing exercise which is needed for bone health in a woman. I wish I had started with short walks sooner, but this was too exhausting. Now it is so much easier. I would never combine two activities in one day. I notice the ache and pain around the mid upper arm is substantially worse. My arm cannot take it. So I don't swim if I am going to have physical therapy that day.

Breast Lymph: The lymph in the breast area after a surgery like this, I would have to say may be expected. It makes perfect sense when so many lymph nodes have been removed, and the fluid needs to and always will travel to the area of least resistance. This has taken months and months and months to improve. But I am pleased to say it continues to move in the right direction. You need to have patience with this symptom and there is nothing you can do to speed it along. I did everything I was instructed to do and nothing made it resolve any faster. I was wearing compression bras that were so binding and constricting at times I wasn't sure if this was the right thing to do. Then I would not wear a bra, just tighter tank tops under my clothing, and this did not help with improving the situation other than the discomfort in my arm seemed less. It's all about finding the right recipe for you. But I believe time was the biggest key.

Patience: Give it T I M E. The amount of time it took me to feel better is going to be different from the amount of time it will take you. For comfort in regards to the arm, I am convinced; compress, relax, elevate, sit up, lie down, it is all a puzzle and it just needs time. Our bodies are amazing and eventually they figure it out and usually adjust over time. It was about the nine- or ten-month mark postsurgery of this magnitude, when I finally noticed my girl looked 'almost' as normal as the other. I also think the lymph fluid will continue to influence the tissue within and around my breast for life. Trying to keep it at a minimum is all we can do, by following the helpful hints outlined in the previous chapter.

Diets: We should always follow a healthy diet. This may be different from person to person. Diabetics have to follow strict guidelines and should. Cardiac patients have dietary guidelines as well. Low-sodium and low-fat diets are always recommended. Trying to maintain a healthy weight is important and seems to always be a challenge, especially as we age. Drinking plenty of water daily for promoting hydration is essential. Just because we drink more water does not mean we retain more water. In fact the opposite is true as it promotes a proper hydrating balance.

New Hobby: Pick up a new hobby or distract yourself with reading or something you really enjoy doing. I was so thankful for the writing inspiration I have had. It provided a very therapeutic outlet for me. Since my retirement, it has been a welcomed alternative. I also did a couple of water colors. I think that is where I might invest more of my time, in painting.

Skin Care: Maintain good hygiene. Apply moisturizer and sunscreen to exposed areas daily. Pay attention to signs of chafing or cracking of the skin. Signs of infection include: rash, itching, redness, pain, skin temperature, increased swelling, fever or flulike symptoms

Refer to suggestions and recommendations earlier in the chapter.

Avoid Extreme Temperatures: Avoid extreme cold that can cause rebound swelling and chafing of skin. On the other hand, extreme heat exposure longer than 15 minutes can cause swelling also. Do not use saunas or hot tubs longer than 15 minutes, use only moderate heat Reconsider using public saunas or hot-tubs at all.

All the above information I think is a common sense approach to our surgical compromise. **You should always follow the plan outlined be your physician, as our course of treatment can vary patient to patient.** I have read all the literature provided me, and consolidated it for the purpose of a basic and sensible approach to be considered for life. Lymph nodes do not rejuvenate or grow back, so it becomes important to take care of the area that is missing them, and promote stimulation with massage to the areas where we still have them.

CHAPTER NINETEEN

WHAT IS MOHS

RETURN DERMATOLOGY APPOINTENT

I remain faithful as I maintained my every-three-months skin checks. I cannot emphasize this enough and I will remain proactive in my skin health care for life. So back to Stanford for a visit in mid-November. There was a fourth-year resident on this visit with my dermatologist. An extra set of eyes never hurts. She was very knowledgeable and confident. I needed a couple of lesions removed, another 'squamous cell carcinoma' was shaved and fully resected from my thigh. I pointed out a small flaky area within my upper left ear and when she saw it she was confident it was a 'basal cell carcinoma.' She gave me a local anesthesia and took a shave biopsy. She was positive I would need Mohs surgery to excise the remainder for adequate borders to be taken and prevent recurrence. Always the goal, prevent recurrence. I had no idea what Mohs surgery was.

I received a phone call once it had been confirmed—yes, basal cell carcinoma. The borders were not clear, and the lesion went deeper than she suspected. Mohs surgery would be the 'proper' course of action. So another appointment was scheduled with the director of Mohs Micrographic and Dermatology Surgery for December 5th, 2017. I had seen her before, as she had done my first melanoma excision with great results. Four years out and one could barely see my previous battle wound as my husband would call it.

What is Mohs?

Mohs Micrographic Surgery (MMS) is an advanced surgical technique designed specifically for the removal of cancers of the skin. Its name is derived from the inventor of the technique, Dr. Fredric Mohs. MMS is based upon the principle of using a microscope to trace skin cancer cells so that the cancer can be completely removed while minimizing the amount of healthy tissue being removed.

The Mohs procedure is used to treat basal and squamous cells carcinomas as well as other rare skin cancers. It is performed in an out-patient setting in one day, under local anesthesia. Of all the treatments for skin cancer, MMS provides the highest cure rate and the greatest conservation of normal tissue, thereby minimizing scarring or recurrence.

The Mohs Procedure

The procedure is as follows: once the local anesthesia is injected to numb the tissue area of concern, they will excise the visible portion of the lesion. Once the skin is removed, she will divide and color-code the sections with dyes and make reference marks on the skin to show the source of these sections. A map of the surgical site is then shown. The undersurface and edges of each section are microscopically examined for evidence of remaining cancer. If the cancer cells are found, the location is marked onto the map and returns to excise more skin, but only precisely where the cancer cells remain. She will continue this process until all cancerous cells are gone and margins are cleared. She does this with such precision and skill. This process can take several hours from start to finish.

My surgeon walked in the room and after a polite greeting the procedure was explained to me. I said, "Good luck, I hope you can get it all in one swipe." She said she definitely could if I wanted to leave with a portion of my ear missing! She was not saying this to be smart-alecky; she went on to explain the importance of preserving as much healthy skin as possible, especially in certain areas of the body. A new skin cancer can pop up in the ear again, and then what? To remove the tip of my ear would be so easy. The real talent of a Mohs micrographic surgeon lies in preserving as much skin in an area that can possibly be spared and be cancer-free, leaving a scar that will barely be visible. The areas that have limited skin for big resections are on the scalp, face, ears, nose, lips, and genitals. So we began with a medication to help me relax, as they explained this procedure might take several hours. Like almost five.

The Mohs procedure began. Her nurse would numb the area of my ear properly and after about fifteen minutes, the doctor entered and proceeded with the first excision. I could not feel anything and I was thankful. I was wondering how this would end up. Would I end up missing the tip of my ear because of this small basal cell if she couldn't get it all? That thought went through my mind, but I quickly dismissed it. As she headed to the lab to evaluate the specimen, she allowed me to get up and go sit with my husband in the waiting room for surgical patients only. The nurse returned about thirty to forty minutes later and said there was still cancer remaining and another excision would be needed. Round two, so back in the room we went. I got adjusted on the table and the doctor entered again, gave me her thoughts. She proceeded to do her thing and reexcised another sample, then off to the lab she went specimen in hand to evaluate microscopically.

Again I rejoined my husband and waited for the news. Another thirty minutes or longer went by and her nurse returned—well, it looked like we are good after this round. She had removed all the cancer. *That is great*, I thought, *she will stitch me up and we will be on our way*. Back in the room we went, I got adjusted again, and the doctor walked in and said, "Okay, we have removed all the cancer. Now I have to close it up by taking a skin graft from either behind your ear or your collar bone." I couldn't believe this— Mohs was new to me. A graft now, for my ear! Are we kidding here? *That lesion was so small*, I thought. Again, I was so thankful for my team of physicians here. I would have no idea how serious this COULD have been had I let this little tiny scaly lesion in my ear go. That is what happens: you let it go and before you know it you have the tip of your ear removed, your lip or your nose. This is called a surgically enhanced deformity for skin cancer.

She inspected both areas carefully and decided she would take the skin graft, which would line the inner upper portion of my ear (called the anterior helix) from my right collar bone area. I said, "Just be sure to recruit skin that doesn't have a freckle or a hair coming out of it." We laughed; I don't need hair growing out of my ear. She assured me it would be fine. Another round of injections to numb the area that the graft site would be taken from by her resident assistant. The doctor proceeded to excise the area of skin she would use to create a graft. She stitched closed the fresh graft site wound and an almost two-inch scar remained. She left the room again and her assistant measured the amount of skin and trimmed it for a graft placement for my ear. The doctor reentered, sat down, and with patience, her zoom lenses, precision and a steady hand, literally needle-pointed a new inner ear graft for me. This part of the Mohs surgery took two and half hours.

This delicate procedure was done with such expertise, again I am amazed at the talent I have been surrounded by. I left with bandage on my ear but my entire ear intact. I was hosting a Christmas coffee at my home on Saturday, so I was appreciative to have yet another procedure behind me. Caring for my ear was delicate. Have you ever tried to place a Band-Aid on the top portion of your ear by yourself? It was sore and so was my collar bone. Another minor adjustment in the simple things I could not do without being cautious. I couldn't just wash my hair and throw it all up in a towel. That could possibly interfere with the new graft. I have to be as patient and delicate with my ear as she was.

She warned me that when I went to change the pressure bandage in three days, it would appear dark in color but not to worry. That once a blood supply was reestablished, it would gradually turn pink. She was right: it turned dark brownish within four to five days and stayed that way until about day ten. It was very important to clean the ear graft site daily and redress it with Vaseline and a Band-Aid. Keeping the graft moistened so as to prevent a scab from forming was extremely important. You do not want to leave it open for air, as it will dry it out. I did this for almost two weeks. I was very compliant with all my instructions.

Now I am almost 4 weeks postsurgery and my ear graft site looks amazing. My right collar bone incision is healing well and will be fading in time. Another scar, all for the sake of medical healing. We have to be good with these decisions. Today I went swimming for the first time since my ear graft, and it felt so good to be back in the water. Therapy I certainly needed again.

Staying diligent cannot be stressed enough in regards to full-skin checks. This will be my course for the rest of my life, and I am okay with that. Melanoma can start as small as a pencil tip, and the earlier it is found the better the outcome. This past year has been valuable in my book of life. **So, I remind you to get a skin check if you are over fifty and never have had one before.**

Behind the Scenes—Breakthroughs

I recently received some additional information from my dermatologist. I mentioned the last time I saw her, early November 2017, I was writing a book. So she remembered this and sent me additional information for me to review. She told me 'to reach out to her' should I need anything. She enclosed a new and beautifully designed booklet that Stanford Health Care and Stanford Cancer Institute collaborated on, titled: *Stopping the most common cancer.* I thanked her for the thoughtful gesture and told her I would read it and summarize some of the amazing behind-the-scene progress that I could share.

I read through the booklet and found it additionally informative. It provided me with insight to some 'behind the scenes' progress being made, from collaborative and multidisciplinary efforts by some of the most brilliant minds at this institution. By them ceaseless efforts are focused on the primary goal of eradicating cancer, first by understanding all they can about the cancer. I find it amazing to learn they were the first to recreate and convert a normal skin cell into basal cell carcinoma in 1997. What this means is they found a way to stimulate a single cell and modify it to become basal cell cancer, all without putting a patient in danger. This enables them to study the cells' response in a multitude of areas and collect crucial data. They are able to understand why it starts, where it starts, how fast it duplicates, when it seems to respond to treatment, and why it becomes resistant to treatment. But that is not all: also what genetic mutations in the family gene pool are contributing to it, etc. This is so much more complicated than I can imagine, but I tried to write it for the purpose of basic understanding here. Their ultimate challenge is to interrupt the cancer and its ability to duplicate, thereby eradicating it before it begins. Their successes or contribution to world-renowned research or breakthroughs will go unnoticed by most of us—the patients. This topic is usually not discussed in the day-to-day appointment settings, and is usually too complicated to grasp. The ongoing research is valuable and can be groundbreaking, because once a melanoma cell breaks off and goes rogue is when the fear sets in for all of us and the death rate surely escalates.

We don't often think of all the people involved who are 'all hands on,' specific to us as the cancer patient. There are so many areas of expertise involved when a skin cancer diagnosis is made. There are geneticists, microbiologists, pathologists, dermatologists, anesthesiologists, nuclear medicine, cutaneous oncology surgeons, and oncologists just to name a few—a truly collaborative effort for the better understanding of our individual diagnosis and treatment needs. The dermatology clinic and its departments provided me a seamless flow from one area to the other regarding my skin cancer needs. Other departments should study how they can successfully achieve this.

New Considerations

There are always new innovations and considerations for trying to prevent and detect skin cancer as early as possible. Awareness, early detection, and treatment of something atypical is always key. Minimizing the risks of skin cancer needs to start at a young age and is multifaceted, and educating adults and youth is important. There are studies suggesting **dietary changes** revealing calcium, vitamin D, and a low-fat diet. Even aspirin can play important roles in preventing melanoma. **Implementing any of these dietary changes should always be reviewed by your physician first.** Good sunscreen habits, just like healthy eating and exercise habits, need to be instilled early in life. While parents may be diligent about the application of sunscreen to their children, once these kids become high school- or college-bound athletes, do they understand the importance of continuing this practice? Especially when athletic fields are being penetrated by UV rays, and most training practices occur in midday hours. There are programs on some college campuses that address and promote the use of sunscreen in athletics departments, but not all.

Almost any major cancer institution has ongoing research within its walls and in various areas of medicine. Of course there will always be ongoing research in the field of genetics. Which is providing more of a personalized approach to improve prediction, prevention, and treatment. Gene sequencing technologies investigating the genetic aspects of skin cancer risk, progression, and response to therapy allows researchers to analyze data that can aid in predicting which new therapies will be most effective for each individual patient. Then this gets way over my head, so we will stop right there.

Since I believe God created us in His image, He already knew whose minds would be able to perform beyond a level of understanding for the rest of us to even comprehend. Thank God there are people smarter than I. Me. Us.

CHAPTER TWENTY

WHAT A JOURNEY

ELEVEN MONTHS CLEAR

The last of my three sets of brain and PET scan were completed in late November and both were negative. How thankful I am once again to hear this news. The month of December can be celebrated to its fullest. I have been moved to every six months for diagnostic surveillance with these. If both scans in June 2018 are negative, then maybe annual scans until I reach the five-year mark may be possible.

My journal entry on January 8, 2018 reads:

> I know this will be a year of recovery still, as last year was all-consuming. But my inner spirit is in new form and I can focus on my Almighty Father and regain some health in my life.

MY PRAYER January 8, 2018

"Let me Glorify Him and be a voice in 2018. Direct me, Lord, for your Greater Purpose, no matter what awaits me. Forgive me for my grumblings. I am sorry and humbled. May my life be transformed to be worthy of Your

Sacrifice and the ransom paid for me. Help me Glorify You this coming year. Amen."

I had written this prayer as I was preparing for my last chapter of this book. But in promising updates, I decided to include it before my updates and conclude with special thoughts.

Lymphedema specialist; February 2018 was my first visit with the lymphedema specialist and it went well. My L-Dex number had actually gone down, as I had been wearing my compression sleeve a bit more. This proves to be effective and aside from the discomfort after wearing the sleeve for several hours, I can remove it. The compression sleeves we can purchase are really beautiful also. As for my blood pressure medication affecting my readings, the answer was no. The L-Dex is specific with unilateral cellular changes. Blood pressure medication does not play a role in this. He told me to keep doing what I was doing, and informed me I had less than a 2 percent chance of lymphedema occurring now if I can make it through the first year without an incident of it. So I will continue to wear my sleeve five hours or so a day until then. I am almost to the year mark in April. Another grateful moment.

Dermatology follow-up; I'm eleven months out and I just had another of my every-three-month follow-up visit with my lead physician. I had one lesion that needed to be removed and I am sure this will be my path for a long time. The pathology results did prove to reveal the lesion on my right shoulder area was a very small melanoma according to the first pathology. But in obtaining a second opinion by another lab for review, they reclassified it because of the size alone as severe dysplastic nevi. This pathology is a higher-risk pathology. It was the size of the smallest circle you can make with your pencil tip. No joke. After a quick conversation with my doctor, a reexcision was done and it was removed in its entirety. I found it doing my full body skin-exam at home. Another scar of my choosing for staying proactive with my diagnosis, which still places me at high-risk for reoccurrence.

I will stay diligent and I encourage you to be with any health issue. My physician provided me with new statistics collected worldwide and reviewed by world-renowned specialists including herself. The outcome of these results will directly affect the treatment plans or protocols for those patients diagnosed with malignant melanoma stage III-A within the next year or so. A treatment plan is always established between the physician and the patient no matter what the statistics prove. So we must always keep that in mind. Because human worry is very real, especially when you hear the word 'cancer' for the very first time. An option for any treatment plan that will aid in 'peace of mind' for us and make us sleep better at night is always a consideration by our physician. And it will usually be mutually agreed upon.

Most insurance companies will indeed adjust their coverage guidelines depending on the latest recommendations by these specialists worldwide who are reviewing the data and setting the new standards. Insurance companies usually tweak their coverage plan based on the recommendations for diagnostics and treatment options per diagnosis from the large cancer associations. NCI or other leading cancer institutions provide the direction for the guidelines insurance companies take their cues from. Meaning: how many PET scans or brain MRIs you can have annually that your insurance will cover under certain diagnosis.

With respect to my arm, I have to tell you the discomfort continues to come and go. I have not had a single day since this surgery was done in April in which I have been pain-free. I have a noticeable concave indentation under my left axilla. While my scars are fading, I have over eighteen inches of reminders on my body related to skin cancer. I can say that while I did not notice improvement on a day-by-day basis, I have noticed improvement as far as the intensity of pain improved as the months passed. Slowly month by month I would notice this month was better than last month and so on. Tylenol is my drug of choice, and only when I really need it. I find I need to give my arm a rest and need to be more disciplined in doing so on a daily basis. We don't realize that our arm hangs with the pull of gravity affecting it every minute of every day. So in order to give it a breather, I need to lie down and rest it, elevated if possible. Try and thwart gravity's pull.

From morning until evening I can feel its effects in my arm. Swimming has been wonderful therapy for me both mentally and physically, and it counters gravity's pull as well. I am so thankful I can swim.

The statistic for my prognosis since the beginning has improved, something I was thrilled to hear on this last visit, and thankful once again for the expert quality care I have received. I was initially diagnosed in January 2017, the second time with malignant melanoma, and I had results of a positive 1/3 sentinel lymph node with the biopsy indicating the smallest amount of melanoma within the lymph node. My five-year survival rate at that time was quoted to be 80 percent—which means I had a 20 percent chance that I could succumb to this ghostly cancer or a complication from it or treatment before the five-year mark. I went on to have the axillary completion surgery done, and had a total of 25 lymph nodes removed, as I have shared with you in this book. But this is when the reality of just how much time is left for me, or any of us with a statistic like that, hit me hard.

In January 2018, with the latest worldwide data and statistics in regards to surveillance monitoring versus immunotherapy and all the risks these drugs posed, the protocol will be changed. Survival rates for my exact situation are now above 90 percent—93 percent to be exact. Wow, this is a huge relief, and shows how important it is to be diligent and compliant with your care and early with detection. She had mentioned that persons with stage III A will no longer be encouraged to consider immunotherapy, but instead offered quarterly surveillance monitoring with ultrasound unless something else should arise. Meaning it won't be discussed as part of the treatment plan.

My declining immunotherapy as part of my treatment plan was God's gift to me. I really believe that. I became physically sick every time I thought about considering it. It was my 'gut' once again talking to me and I listened to it. I am thankful I understand a bit more about medicine than the average layman and being a nurse practitioner has been my calling. I did officially tender my resignation in early August to the college, which was extremely difficult for me to do. I had too much on my plate and maybe if I had been ten years younger, I would have continued down this path. Even writing this book has had its physical challenges, for example with typing that requires a bent elbow. Having my arm bent for an extended period of time causes discomfort to say the least. I had many rest periods in between my writing, and I will be glad once it is completed. I will wait and listen for signs or inspiration on where my path will take me next. But this twofold journey this past year in 2017 I would not trade for anything. It was all meant to be.

So after almost one year, my journey with its unsteady footing through the peaks and valleys a cancer diagnosis can bring, I can honestly say; I know I did not get through this alone. My loved ones, family, friends, and physicians were all in this with me. I could not have appreciated them more. They loved me, supported me, prayed for me, and most likely I have experienced medical healing. But while some may have felt the heaviness in their heart to watch me go through this, I would soon recognize, no one could share the burden, give me courage, or alleviate my worry and fear on any given day as much as they would have wanted to. I had to help myself and I was rewarded with an amazing discovery.

With all of my scars, twenty-five lymph nodes or 'pearls' removed and a concave indent under my left arm is where this journey for now ends. The emotional turmoil which was unwelcomed and unexpected in contemplating my treatment options is when I noticed the physical symptoms of fear and uncertainty appear. That must have been when the reality of the 'cancer' diagnosis set in, and I felt so emotionally ill-prepared to handle it all. I do not know if there is anything else I could have tried, besides my spiritual nurturing, which would have alleviated my fear associated with such a profound diagnosis. Surely there are welcomed distractions for the moment like: activities, exercise, yoga, and meditation are but a few. There are many emotions experienced with a hefty challenge of any kind. My spiritual nourishment was refueling my emotional and physical fatigue 24/7, so as to reset the balance which can be lost in the journey. The balance for emotional wellness in all areas of life is vitally important. None of us know how long the struggle will be, or if a new challenge is just over the next peak. The trek for emotional wellness may take days, weeks, months or even years to figure out. Figuring it out became a necessity and one of my goals.

All of the unknown factors, in hefty challenges- medical or otherwise, can yield to fear within us. And when the element of fear is experienced, and we persevere through the trial, our 'inner Holy Spirit' becomes our own hero. The baby steps trying to mature in my faith, which engaged me in a relationship with my God, proved He would be the ONLY ONE who could and would prepare me to defeat that scary element of fear for me. It was only through my time spent with Him, and all the Holy Spirit moments I would encounter, that filled me with an 'inner peace' as my reward. His Perfect Peace as I sat for a visit is indescribable. Suddenly a new normal is welcomed and life feels natural again, with Him in it. What an amazing discovery in a journey of uncertainty and it all started with one- little- baby- step.

If you are in the midst of an awful fight with cancer, any kind of cancer, I would recommend the book *The Strength You Need*. You will find your Hope, which will give you the strength to get through another day.

Just as I am not a dermatologist, I am not a theologian either. Again, there are experts who write on this subject daily and have devoted their entire careers to studying medicine, preaching, or sharing the Gospel. I will only do what I can do. That is to share what I have learned in both of these areas, the both that may affect life and death. My intertwined journey that brought me to write this as a testimony in both arenas I would only hope to one day share with you. I needed baby steps in building my new relationship with God and did this with my daily readings. I just started one day. Suddenly new discoveries were revealed to me, all impactful witness of the Holy Spirit's presence. He blessed Kendyl and me with visions that were powerful and while only experienced by us, were meant to be shared with you.

Seeing His face in the clouds on the perfect 'first swim' day was a day I thought something amazing was yet to happen. My heart was bursting that day with joy, and I still did not know what awaited me. And it just continued. My request asking Jesus to be with me on my 'big surgery' day will forever remain the most profound and blessed day of my life. First in my public declaration of my love for Him, He fulfilled my desire to have Him with me and then validated His Presence through a vision while Kendyl was in deep prayer for me. All the while keeping a Promise He makes to all who seek Him out. For I was not alone. Again such an amazing reward; I felt I received the Gold medal. Well—I still get chills as I recall it all vividly.

I then continued to nurture my relationship with God, just as you nurture a relationship with a loved one. If you want it to be a healthy and loving one, you must first respect it, and then invest time in it. Plant the seed and watch it blossom into the unexpected. That is exactly what happened to me: it blossomed into the unexpected!

I would encourage to start with the NIV Bible and a good daily devotional, like *Jesus Calling*. Maybe consider going to church with a friend. If you are on the fence in regards to Creation, the book I mentioned earlier, *The Language of God*, is an excellent read. It is for those who would appreciate seeing how one man trying to refute and disprove the notion of creation comes to be a believer in his ten years on a groundbreaking project and discovers instead that science and Christianity reinforce each other's existence. These are interesting food-for-thought comments I share below.

Spiritual Pearl ~ Eleven

Now the debate about 'faith' or higher power has been going on for centuries. There will always be opposition to derail any belief, especially in regards to the existence of a Supreme Being. This topic will always be popular to those who need to be so convincing that He doesn't exist. A topic that will never go away. Opposing curiosities or beliefs will forever be of this world. He exists, He doesn't exist. Right versus wrong, meaning no absolute truth, only 'ethical' decisions that are relative. Truth that is relative. I know what truth to me means. Is there good versus evil? We know bad things happen by bad people: does this mean we believe in evil? Does this always mean there is a 'Bad Place'? If so, then we must believe there is the opposite of evil, or good. And does 'good' mean there is a Heaven? For those who refute the existence of God, they must have their reasons. But is there a seed of fear in that He 'might' exist? Or that 'believers' will interfere with them attaining their agendas? Otherwise, I agree with Dr. Collins: why does there need to be an argument in the first place? I don't know why it is so important or matters so much to them. What is in the atheist agenda that provides hope for a better life? If you do not believe in God because 'we' say He doesn't exist, for this reason and that reason you will live a more complete and joyous life. Is this the agenda? Just because that is their truth?

But the agenda of the atheist opponent, the believer or Christian, is very clear. It is to be a disciple of the Lord and spread the Word or Good News of forgiveness and salvation for an Eternal Life. Through Jesus Christ. The perfect Christmas gift to the World. Why would I look the other way and stay silent when this Gift is the best thing to have ever happened to mankind?

The Last Holy Spirit Moment ~ Seven

IN CONCLUSION

It was actually on January 21, 2018, after I attended worship service and came home to prepare my last entry for this book, when I felt the Holy Spirit aiding me once again on the avenue of scripture to conclude my medical and spiritual journey. I think how appropriate that my journaling would begin on a beautiful, pristine spring morning and conclude on a beautiful, pristine winter morning.

In reflecting all that has transpired this past year—from the moment the physician delivered the news of melanoma making its way into my lymph nodes, the five-year survival rate associated with it, to the ripple effect it would have on my life trying to defeat it, I have never had a more challenging and difficult year—that I felt so richly blessed. For the cancer 'pearls' had been clearly woven into the most incredible spiritual journey of my life. In one simple moment, all of the trials in this year's challenge would impact and transform my entire future.

The ripple effect, as I chose to call it, is everything I shared with you here, in this raw, exposed medical and spiritual trek I have persevered through. With excellent medical care and a spiritual awaking to help. As a provider, I never could appreciate the day in and day out struggles when a diagnosis becomes a sudden challenge for a patient. Now as the patient and still living it, I can empathize—completely. We do not go home with you to make sure you are doing okay, or make sure you have everything you need.

Nor do we truly understand what life is like in 'your shoes' with 'your circumstances.' The real life story and behind-the-scene moments in the life of a patient became very real to me. All the little details we as providers never hear about, or think about when you come in for an appointment with us. We may sympathize, but we don't live it with you.

I'm thankful I chose my something to- *lean* on, *rely* on, *trust* on, and *hope* on. So many special people, My Jesus, and The Trinity saw me through. But as I sat in worship this morning, I realized once again the Holy Spirit was speaking directly to me and laid out the last scripture I would quote for the conclusion of this book before me. So I thank Pastor Mark and I write today—this final chapter—which once again is perfectly pertinent in its timing.

"When Jesus called the Twelve together, he gave them power and authority to drive out all the demons and cure diseases, and he sent them out to proclaim the kingdom of God, and heal the sick."

LUKE 9:1–2

His Word has spanned the globe for centuries, first by the Chosen Twelve, His disciples. Who with obedient hearts fulfilled His command and kept their promise to Jesus until their last breath. His Truth will live on and be faithfully shared by all those from the past, those here and now, and those in the future with obedient hearts, to be the voices to complete His work while on this earth, as He has instructed us to do.

So it is with an obedient heart that I first recognize this book would never have been possible for me to complete had the proclamation of the kingdom of God not first penetrated the depth of my soul. And with the renewing and maturing of my faith through the power of the Holy Spirit, and all the material provided and unveiled before me by Him, would I be able to share my journey with you.

A journey that has always been twofold. First, to help people become more aware of skin cancers, in particular malignant melanoma cancer and all that it can potentially bring with it. **If you have any concerns regarding lesions on your body, do not hesitate to have them checked out.** I hope my trek brought you some encouragement, especially if your journey is difficult. Remember you need to replenish your strength and courage daily, for the challenge can feel overwhelming at times. Daily refueling is so important when fatigue is ever present. So what and how will you choose to lean, rely, trust, or hope on while trying to accomplish this? Secondly, the interwoven spiritual transformation of my mind from being a 'believer' to the overwhelming joy I experienced within my heart, with being a 'believer in a relationship' with my Heavenly Father. Both of these journeys inspired by the Holy Spirit, and shared in the hopes of saving just one life.

This strand of 'Pearls' I mentioned before signifying the Trinity embodies His church—which is a MASTERPIECE created only by God. It has no limit to its length, is a priceless strand, and will never be sold. It will be my reminder every time I wear my strand of pearls around my neck. Maybe the next time you wear a strand you will feel differently, as it may be just the reminder you need to sustain a spiritual awareness of the Trinity as they grace your neck. Wear a strand and see how you feel.

He has no Equal. My prayer is for all of our hearts to be sealed with His Grace, Mercy, Wisdom, and Love. So when our time comes and we may bow down before Him, we know with certainty we will see the face of God. For this is the truth in the 'Hope' that awaits us.

So I will be one voice for Him while I walk on my journey toward heaven. My scars will forever be my battle wounds, but even those are fading now. What will remain steadfast in me forever is the experience of learning patience, trusting completely, listening intently, being still in the moments, and welcoming Him for a visit while loving, respecting, and nurturing a relationship I hold dear. I learned to recognize my scars as forever reminders of the amazing 'pearls' I discovered with my medical healing and spiritual journey, as I allowed Him to take full residence in the center of my heart.

So from *Scars to Pearls*, what a beautiful canvas He had a hand in.

ACKNOWLEDGEMENTS

I would like to give a special thank-you to my dermatologist for taking the time to read my book and provide me with feedback on the skin cancer medical content in this book. I'm not sure if I can properly convey just how much that meant to me. You are such a skilled and knowledgeable physician and just a wonderful human being. I thank God for having our paths cross.

It is with much appreciation I thank Pastor Mark Krieger for reading *Scars to Pearls* and guiding me through the history of the Bible and The Holy Trinity with such patience. His passion for God and broad knowledge in theology provided understanding and affirmation to my baby steps while on my spiritual journey.

Foreword Written for

SCARS TO PEARLS

In *Scars to Pearls*, Lita Worthington shares her personal story with malignant melanoma skin cancer. Being a nurse practitioner herself, Lita has to now be the patient and experiences the surgical recovery hardships that can only be understood firsthand. In this journey, she has profound experiences that can only be explained by God. God working behind the scenes through people and circumstances that provided her and loved ones comfort through visions and dreams. Lita felt God's encouragement through Scripture verses and Holy Spirit moments that she shares with us. *Scars to Pearls* brings a new alert to skin cancer awareness, and her spiritual journey will cause you to look at your own life differently.

~ MARK KRIEGER, LEAD PASTOR, MODESTO COVENANT CHURCH

I am amazed by the depth and fluidity of your writing. It is very intimate and personal. The Holy Spirit clearly is working in you like never before. It's hard for me to settle on what I am most grateful for, your physical healing or your spiritual awakening. Having walked this journey with you, I have deepened my love for you and for the Lord. He comforted you when only He could. He guided us to blessed physicians. He made alive His Word to nourish and strengthen our souls. In the depths of the fear and sadness that this last year took us through, we experienced in vivid colors 'the peace that surpasses all understanding.' And you Lita are my hero, my inspiration, and my girl. I'll love you for eternity... through our Lord and Savior Jesus Christ.

~ SCOTT, HUSBAND

CPSIA information can be obtained
at www.ICGtesting.com
Printed in the USA
LVHW08s0430150918
590115LV00001B/1/P